21 SECRETS FOR A HEALTHY GUT

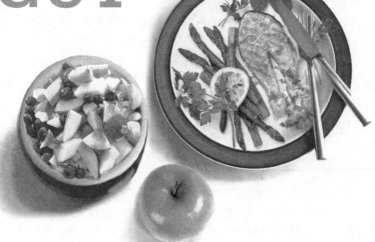

SILOAM

Most CHARISMA HOUSE BOOK GROUP products are available at special quantity discounts for bulk purchase for sales promotions, premiums, fund-raising, and educational needs. For details, write Charisma House Book Group, 600 Rinehart Road, Lake Mary, Florida 32746, or telephone (407) 333-0600.

21 SECRETS FOR A HEALTHY GUT edited by Siloam
Published by Siloam
Charisma Media/Charisma House Book Group
600 Rinehart Road
Lake Mary, Florida 32746
www.charismahouse.com

Cover design by Justin Evans

For more information on Siloam, visit
www.charismahouse.com.

Library of Congress Cataloging-in-Publication Data:
21 secrets for a healthy gut / [edited by] Siloam.
    pages cm
  Summary: "Health begins in your gut. Prevention is a main felt need for
people who want to live full lives and be around for their families. Gut
health is essential to wellness and a high quality of life. With the success of
the Bible Cure series and the popularity of healthy living, the market is right
for simplified, proven ways to maintain great health, a balanced life, and
long life. This book will explore various remedies, diets, detoxes, superfoods,
supplements, vitamins, and treatments to heal the gut--the gastrointestinal
system of the body. Proper function of this area of the body is key to
healing just about any lifestyle disease we are facing in the twenty-first
century. This book will also explore causes and cures for inflammation, poor
absorption, constipation, leaky gut, Crohn's disease, wheat belly, wheat brain,
IBS, candida, GERD, ulcerative colitis, celiac disease, and more. Expert
contributions from Don Colbert, Janet Maccaro, Cherie Calbom, Reginald
Cherry, and others"-- Provided by publisher.
  ISBN 978-1-62998-210-6 (paperback) -- ISBN 978-1-62998-586-2
(e-book)
  1. Gastrointestinal system--Diseases--Alternative treatment--Popular works.
2. Self-care, Health--Popular works. I. Title: Twenty one secrets for a
healthy gut.
  RC806.A13 2015
  616.3'3--dc23
                       2015008583

Portions of this book were previously published by Siloam as *The Juice
Lady's Big Book of Juices and Smoothies* by Cherie Calbom, ISBN: 978-1-
62136-030-8, copyright © 2013; *Answers for the 4-A Epidemic* by Joseph A.

Cannizzaro, ISBN: 978-1-61638-484-5, copyright © 2012; *The Bible Cure* by Reginald Cherry, ISBN: 978-0-88419-535-1, copyright © 1998; *Eat This and Live* by Don Colbert, ISBN: 978-1-59979-519-5, copyright © 2009; *The Bible Cure for Candida and Yeast Infections* by Don Colbert, ISBN: 978-0-88419-743-0, copyright © 2001; *The Bible Cure for Weight Loss* by Don Colbert, ISBN: 978-1-61638-616-0, copyright © 2013; *The Bible Cure for Irritable Bowel Syndrome* by Don Colbert, ISBN: 978-1-59979-736-6, copyright © 2002; *The Bible Cure for Heartburn and Indigestion* by Don Colbert, ISBN: 978-0-88419-651-8, copyright © 1999; *Jump Start!* by David Herzog, ISBN: 978-1-62136-595-4, copyright © 2014; *Natural Health Remedies* by Janet Maccaro, ISBN: 978-1-59185-897-3, copyright © 2006; *30 Quick Tips for Better Health* by Don VerHulst, ISBN: 978-1-62136-210-4, copyright © 2013; *Do This and Live Healthy* by Don VerHulst, ISBN: 978-1-61638-826-3, copyright © 2012.

15 16 17 18 19 — 9876543

Printed in the United States of America

CONTENTS

YOUR GUT: THE CENTER OF IT ALL

Y**OU ARE WHAT** you eat" is likely a statement you heard growing up. If your mother uttered that phrase, she may have been trying to persuade you to finish your vegetables. Still, Mom was right—to a degree. The statement is more accurately phrased: "You are what you eat *and* what you are able to absorb." You can eat all the lima beans and green peas in the world, but unless your body can absorb the nutrients in these vegetables, they don't do you any good!

Like many other diseases in our culture, gastrointestinal disorders are on the rise. From ailments as common as heartburn to more serious problems, such as ulcers, acid reflux disease, and irritable bowel syndrome (IBS), your digestive system is under attack. In a manner similar to the immune system, the digestive system is your first line of defense against harmful agents in the world around you. All the nutrients your body takes in pass through the digestive system. It is therefore crucial to maintain gastrointestinal (GI) health and protect your body from attack.

You may think your digestive system's primary function is to digest food. True, yet the digestive system does much more for the body. There are four major processes of digestion that will be helpful to understand for protecting your health:

1. First, your body must *digest* food. You must take in the food and break it down into various tiny components the body can use for energy.

2. Your body must eliminate waste. It can't use every molecule of food, so it must sort out and remove substances that are not helpful or good.

3. Your body must *absorb* nutrients. Without absorbing the nutrition available in that food, you will literally starve to death.

4. Your body must *normalize* its balance of "good" bacteria in your intestines. Otherwise known as *flora*, these good bacteria must be present in the colon for your body to function properly.

All four of these processes must be operating successfully to prevent or treat gastrointestinal disorders. And this all takes place in the gut, sometimes called the "second brain." You can't enjoy the benefits of good health without a healthy diet, proper digestion, and avoiding the foods that can lead to such gastrointestinal issues as irritable bowel diseases, inflammatory issues, poor food absorption, constipation, or leaky gut syndrome.

This is why a proper diet is so essential to a healthy gut—and a healthy body. Digestion of food begins almost as soon as you eat it, but it only takes place in the presence of enzymes. The key enzymes for digestive health include 1) amylase enzymes, which break down carbohydrates; 2) lipase, which break down fats; and 3) proteolytic enzymes, which break down proteins. A deficiency in any of these enzymes can result in a host of uncomfortable digestive problems, such as gas, bloating, diarrhea, or constipation.

Without the proper amounts of enzymes necessary for digestion to take place, particles of food will pass through the body undigested and create these difficulties. However, a more serious effect of an enzyme deficiency is fatigue. If problems occur at the digestive stage, the body won't break down the food to the stage where the system absorbs it and provides nutrition to the cells. Consequently, your energy sources get quickly depleted, leaving you feeling tired all the time.

One unusual ailment that is in early stages of research is the aforementioned leaky gut syndrome. This occurs when the proteolytic enzymes that digest protein are either not present in sufficient quantities or are not functioning correctly. Leaky gut syndrome is believed to take place when larger protein molecules that have missed being properly digested earlier in the digestive tract migrate to the "gut" (small intestine), where they are absorbed. This absorption in an inappropriate area creates an immunological response from the body and can cause such immune-related problems as allergies or arthritis.

This syndrome is just one example of the need to pay attention to good gut health. If you have heard the talk about such topics as gluten-free diets, probiotics, and detoxification, and passed it off as a fad or health extremists' propaganda, think again. The information in this simple guide can help you move toward improved gut health. Your body will thank you.

Chapter 1

GLUTEN-FREE ZONE

ELIAC SPRUE DISEASE only affects about 1 percent of the American population. This condition stems from an allergic reaction to gluten, which is a protein found mainly in wheat products. The allergic reaction in the gut damages the tiny villi that line the small intestine. When this happens, the body can no longer properly absorb both fats and carbohydrates. Symptoms of celiac sprue are similar to those of irritable bowel syndrome, and can include things such as stomach cramps or pains, constipation, or mucus in the stool. However, there is one major exception: Celiac sprue will cause excessive diarrhea and lead to significant weight loss. Treating it means eliminating all gluten-containing foods and products from the diet. In addition to wheat, grains such as oats, barley, and rye also contain gluten.

With such a small percentage of people affected by this disease, skeptics may scoff at the idea of considering a gluten-free diet. However, there are reasons other than celiac sprue to examine this option, starting with the foods so popular in the traditional American diet. While modern food processing systems remove fiber and many vitamins from the breads, pastas, cereals, and other starches we consume, the problem may not be limited to the refining process. The wheat itself may be the culprit. Renowned cardiologist William Colbert Davis, MD, believes foods made with or containing wheat are the number one reason Americans are fat and suffering from diabetes—and all the digestive and other health problems stemming from obesity.

In order to increase crop production, modern wheat strains have been hybridized, crossbred, and genetically altered by agricultural scientists.[1] As a result, modern strains of wheat have a higher quantity of genes for gluten proteins that are associated with celiac disease.[2] Modern wheat also contains a starch called amylopectin A, which raises blood sugar levels more than virtually any other carbohydrate.[3] In addition, wheat is an appetite stimulant, making you want more and more food.[4] It is

1

also considered addictive. Approximately 30 percent of all people who stop eating wheat products experience withdrawal symptoms, such as extreme fatigue, mental fog, irritability, inability to function at work, and depression.[5] The addictive nature of wheat, coupled with the fact that it triggers exaggerated blood sugar and insulin responses, sets your body up to pack on the pounds.

Proper Enzymes

As a protein, gluten requires a particular enzyme, DPP4, to break it down successfully within the human body. This enzyme is also involved in the digestion of milk and milk products, all of which contain casein. With children and adults in whom DPP4 does not function fully, their bodies do not fully break down the gluten or casein. The result is peptides (partial proteins) that mimic the chemical composition of opiates or endorphins and cause similar feelings to occur when they reach the brain.

The pleasure of spaciness and sense of intoxication this often produces makes it hard to give up gluten, particularly for children. In fact, kids often crave processed carbohydrates. These are the very foods that feed the pathogens in the gut, and can interfere with the process necessary for the body to detoxify itself. Naturally, children and adults who get used to a diet heavy in dairy products, processed carbohydrates (breads, cakes, cookies, chips, cereals, pastas), and sugar don't want to change their food preferences. Failing to change an unhealthy diet, though, will simply prolong the pain.

Particularly with children, when it comes to distress in the digestive tract, most autistic kids, ADHD kids, and severe asthmatics—including all severely allergic children—will benefit from a diet that is strictly free of gluten (grains) and dairy (casein). The removal of these foods provides the foundation of dietary interventions for such disorders. Additional changes will always be needed for more complete improvement, but the standard initial dietary intervention is a gluten-free/casein-free (GF/CF) diet. No single diet solves everything or applies across the board, yet this particular one has shown the most promising results.

The reason? As long ago as 1971 researcher M. S. Goodwin documented abnormal brain responses to gluten. A decade later other researchers showed that children who maintained a GF/CF diet showed improved cognition, language, and behavior. It is now believed that certain peptides (amino acid chains) from gluten and casein can bind to opioid receptors in the brain, causing a powerful effect on behavior. Symptoms include "zoning out," aggression, self-abuse, and either constipation or diarrhea.

The Gluten-Free/Casein-Free Diet

Basic List of Foods Allowed

(This list must be modified to accommodate specific allergies and food sensitivities.)

- Almond milk and other nut milks
- Amaranth
- Beans and legumes (prepared from dry or unseasoned canned)
- Beef
- Buckwheat
- Chicken
- Coconut milk
- Corn flour
- Eggs
- Fish
- Fruits (all plain fresh or frozen, most canned; avoid dried)
- Fruit juices (plain)
- Lamb
- Meats (fresh or frozen, plain)
- Millet
- Nuts (all types, unflavored)
- Oats, if gluten-free
- Oils (all types)
- Quinoa
- Rice
- Rice milk
- Potatoes (fresh, plain)
- Seeds (all types)
- Shellfish
- Soy milk
- Turkey
- Vegetables (all unprocessed)

Basic List of Foods to Avoid

- Baby foods (prepackaged)
- Baked goods (bagels, biscuits, bread, bread crumbs, bread stuffing, cake, chow mein noodles, cookies, crackers, croissants, croutons, doughnuts, ice cream cones, muffins, pancakes, pastry, pies, pita bread, pizza, pretzels, rolls, tortillas, waffles)
- Barley, barley grass
- Beverage mixes
- Bologna
- Bouillon, instant
- Bran (except rice)
- Brewer's yeast
- Broth, prepackaged
- Bulgur
- Butter
- Candy (most)
- Cereals (most)
- Cheeses
- Chicken nuggets (and any breaded meat or fish)
- Cold cuts
- Couscous
- Cream sauces
- Durum wheat
- Farina
- Flour
- Custard, pudding
- Gum (most)
- Hot dogs
- Ice cream, ice milk
- Kasha
- Kefir
- Marzipan
- Mashed potatoes
- Matzo semolina
- Milk (all types, from animal sources)
- Milk chocolate
- Muesli
- Nougat
- Pasta, noodles, macaroni, spaghetti
- Potato chips
- Rye
- Salad dressings (creamy or commercially prepared)
- Sausage
- Semolina
- Sour cream
- Soy sauce
- Sprouted wheat or barley
- Syrups
- Tabbouleh
- Teriyaki sauce
- Triticale
- Vegetables in sauces
- Wheat germ
- Wheat grass
- Yogurt
- Zwieback

Note: You would be surprised at the hiding places of gluten and casein in prepackaged foods. For example, canned fish and prepared rice products may contain milk protein. Package banners such as "dairy free" and "nondairy" do not mean casein-free, only that the package contains less than 0.5 percent milk by weight—which translates into as much casein as whole milk.

These peptides appear to cause trouble for ASD (autism spectrum disorder) kids because of improper digestion and gut inflammation, common problems in this population. The Autism Research Institute of San Diego tracks the efficacy of many treatments. Over 60 percent of its respondents report improvement from dietary intervention.

Whether you have recognized the need for a better diet for yourself, or see the need to improve your children's well-being, health enthusiasts and wise shoppers must recognize that not all gluten-free and casein-free foods are the same. After the GF/CF diet spread through many natural foods communities, companies adjusted by marketing prepared foods that may well be gluten- and casein-free but are full of sugar, altered fats, and proteins. Learn what you are avoiding, and learn to read labels; many gluten-free breads, crackers, pastas, and baking products are available from reputable companies.

Food Allergies

The modern increase in food allergies is another reason to consider a low- or gluten-free diet. A food allergy is an autoimmune system response to a certain food or a deficiency of an enzyme needed to digest a certain food. Among the symptoms of such allergies are irritability, headaches, itchy or watery eyes, gas, constipation, sinus problems, nausea, brain fog, or ringing in the ears. They are fast becoming as common as a cold or flu because of all of the chemically altered, injected, sprayed, and dyed foods that Americans ingest on a daily basis.

Add to that stress, lack of sleep, and enzyme deficiency from foods that are zapped by microwave preparation, and the situation has grown worse. Other causes include inherited food sensitivities, MSG, sulfites and nitrates, and food additives that are added to enhance color and flavor and cause a myriad of problems for sensitive individuals.

There's more than your gut at stake here. Two examples:

+ Headaches

    Common in an era of increased stress and tension, headaches seem to occur most frequently in A-type personalities—people who are highly goal-oriented perfectionists who demand a great deal from themselves and those around them. There are two basic types of headaches: those resulting from stress and tension, and those brought on by a physical cause. Stress control is the way to go when it comes to breaking the headache cycle. Food allergies are among the physical causes of headaches. Other causes are oral contraceptives, a sluggish liver, poor circulation or posture, too much caffeine, and magnesium deficiency.

+ Gallbladder problems

    Gallbladder disease is an inflammation of the gallbladder caused by saturated bile known as gallstones. These ailments are on the rise in America because of poor diets filled with sugars and low in fiber, leading to poor digestion. Over twenty million Americans have gallstones and/or gallbladder inflammation known as cholecystitis. The majority of sufferers are women, who account for 75 percent of the cases.[6]

    The gallbladder helps digest fats by producing bile. If the gallbladder bile fluids become saturated with cholesterol, solid crystals form and eventually become gallstones. The key plan of attack is to increase bile solubility to reduce cholesterol levels. In addition, bile flow needs to be increased to aid the gallbladder in expelling small stones. Symptoms include pain in the upper right abdomen during an attack, nausea, cold sweats, belching, anxiety, and others. Some people report that the symptoms made them feel as if they were having a heart attack. The pain becomes more intense as the stones enlarge.

Again, food allergies are a cause of gallbladder problems, as are such factors as chronic indigestion stemming from excessive refined sugar and dairy products, eating too many fried and fatty foods, a sedentary lifestyle, and birth control pills and estrogen replacement therapy, which cause an increase in cholesterol production.

Chapter 2

PROBIOTICS

PROBIOTICS APPEARS ON multiple products in supermarkets these days. This class of healthy foods and supplements has migrated into the fad category, with labels sometimes ranging beyond the reasonable. However, don't let the hype mislead you or prompt you to question their value. Probiotics are simply foods and supplements that contain live "good" bacteria similar to those found in a healthy human gut. Along with prebiotics, which are foods that promote the growth of beneficial bacteria (legumes, peas, soy beans, garlic, onions, leeks, and chives), probiotics can help rebuild and nourish the gut lining.

Probiotics are live microorganisms thought to be healthy for the host organism. Probiotics are commonly consumed as part of fermented foods with specially added active live cultures—such as in yogurt—or as dietary supplements. They help ensure healthy digestive conditions and healthy bacterial flora. Whether foods or supplements, they will put friendly bacteria into your system that will trigger your metabolism, improve digestion, and help cleanse your body.

If you are battling any kind of digestive or intestinal problem, probiotics are a must for your health-building toolbox. These gastrointestinal defenders are crucial in keeping your immune defense in good working order. They consist mainly of lactobacillus acidophilus and lactobacillus bifidus and produce volatile fatty acids, which provide metabolic energy. In addition, they help you digest food and amino acids, produce certain vitamins, and most importantly, make your lower intestine mildly acidic. This helps inhibit the growth of bad bacteria such as *E. coli*, which has caused serious illnesses in recent years.

A word to women: Probiotic supplementation is essential in your fight against candida or any fungal infection because of the antifungal properties that these defenders possess. According to Dr. James F. Balch in his best-selling book, *Prescription for Nutritional Healing*, the flora in a healthy colon should consist of at least 85 percent lactobacilli and 15 percent coliform bacteria.[1] The typical colon bacteria count today is the reverse, which has resulted in gas, bloating, intestinal and systemic toxicity, constipation, and malabsorption of nutrients, making it a perfect environment for the overgrowth of candida.

By adding probiotics—that is, lactobacillus acidophilus and lactobacillus bifidus supplements—to your system, you will return your intestinal flora to a healthier balance and eliminate problems of intestinal flora imbalance. If you are on antibiotic therapy, it is vitally important that you supplement your digestive tract with probiotics, because antibiotic use destroys your healthy bowel flora along with harmful bacteria. Both lactobacillus acidophilus and lactobacillus bifidus promote proper digestion, help normalize bowel function, and prevent gas and candida overgrowth. This in turn keeps immunity high.

As a dietary supplement, take one capsule with a meal twice daily. Children under four should take one-half capsule with a meal twice daily. If the child cannot swallow the capsule, simply open it and sprinkle it in juice or on food. Also, eating organic, plain yogurt with active probiotic cultures can help reintroduce balance to your system.

"Good" Bacteria

Modern society has transformed "bacteria" into a synonym for "germ," "disease," or "unhealthy." Be careful to avoid this simplistic stereotyping. While problems in enzyme production will affect your body's digestive functions, other potential difficulties can occur when the balance between "good" and "bad" bacteria in the intestines is disrupted. It seems strange to some people that any sort of bacteria could be beneficial, but it is true. God created these good bacteria—also known as flora—to live in our intestines and overwhelm the bad bacteria that can cause infections or other serious illnesses. There are over four hundred different species of helpful flora naturally residing in the colon.

Even the term describing this type of bacteria is fascinating. The literal meaning of that word has special significance to people who understand that God created our bodies to be the temple, or dwelling place, for His Holy Spirit. *Probiotic* means "pro life," or "promoting life." For example, when you inadvertently drink polluted water that contains harmful bacteria, the probiotic bacteria in your digestive system attack the foreign invader, literally promoting life in your body.

Another function of the flora is to keep the normal yeast levels of the intestines in balance. If this gets out of hand, especially in women, commonly recurring yeast infections will occur. An underlying cause of these infections is an insufficient amount of good bacteria in the colon. Additionally some forms of bacteria in the intestines assist in the production of enzymes, one of which is lactase, an enzyme that breaks down the lactose sugars in milk and dairy products. One potential cause of lactose intolerance, then, could be a deficiency in the bacteria that produce lactase.

Why Antibiotics Can be Harmful

A discussion of probiotics needs to touch on their opposite: antibiotics. Many health experts call the overprescribing of antibiotics and their use in animal feed and other sources a serious health problem, since it is creating strains of super-resistant bacteria. Still, the common misconception many people have that all bacteria are bad may lead them to think that antibiotics therefore must be good. But take into account the earlier definition of probiotic bacteria. If *probiotic* means to promote life, then what might *antibiotic* mean? Yes, antibiotics are literally "against life," most commonly against the life of bad bacteria. However, when you ingest an antibiotic into your body, it doesn't know the difference between good bacteria and bad bacteria. It kills them all.

Sometimes a round of antibiotics is necessary to knock out a bacterial infection or a case of pneumonia, but if you have taken antibiotics for any reason, you should consider recolonizing your intestines with the good flora that were wiped out by the antibiotics.

The following substances may be taken to restore a normal balance of bacteria in the intestines:

- Arabinogalactan, 250 milligrams (mg) per day
- Fructooligosaccharides, 100 mg per day
- Lactobacillus, 150 mg per day

You may say to yourself, "I haven't needed to take an antibiotic for years!" Even if that is the case, it is a good idea to recolonize your intestines periodically. You may not have been prescribed an antibiotic by your doctor, but have you eaten chicken lately? Poultry, among other animals raised for America's food supply, are regularly treated with antibiotics. They remain in the poultry's system right up until you take that first bite. Every bite thereafter slowly kills off the good bacteria in your colon.

For these reasons, it is important to supplement your digestive system with probiotics, as well as enzymes and fiber, particularly that found in konjac root. A word about the latter: As noted in chapter 1, the body cannot use everything you eat and must eliminate the "leftovers." This is why it is important to eat more fiber, which helps in the elimination process. The fibers that are most helpful are water soluble, which means they are able to absorb the water from the waste product.

Konjac root is commonly used in Japan and may contribute significantly to their health, giving the Japanese the longest average life span in the world. An unusual water-soluble fiber called glucomannan is formulated from this konjac root. The most amazing fact about glucomannan is the sheer amount of water it can absorb: *two hundred times* its own weight. This means that small amounts of it can have a major impact in absorbing watery waste in your intestines.

Another significant function of glucomannan is that it aids in the absorption of cholesterol, all the while creating a feeling of fullness in the stomach as it soaks up water and expands. It contains no calories and suppresses the appetite because of its volume. For these reasons, the konjac root is becoming important as a weight loss supplement. An additional benefit of glucomannan is its ability to regulate blood sugar. Through its immediate absorption of water, it slows down the absorption of sugar into the bloodstream; it can therefore be essential in leveling out the spikes and drops in blood sugar that are so harmful, especially to diabetics.

Chapter 3

THE CANDIDA CURE

CANDIDA, CANDIDIASIS, OR the yeast syndrome is simply an overgrowth of yeast, usually in the intestinal tract and other tissues. In women, painful yeast infections that infect the vagina can cause premenstrual syndrome (PMS) and reduced sex drive. Such overgrowth can also occur in the gastrointestinal tract, causing heartburn, indigestion, abdominal bloating, cramps, constipation or diarrhea, nausea, and gas.

Excessive yeast overgrowth is also related to environmental sensitivities and illnesses that heighten sensitivities to foods, chemicals such as smoke, chemical odors from carpets and fabrics, and auto exhaust. Yet yeast is everywhere (food, air, land), so avoiding exposure is impossible. As a matter of fact, yeast normally lives in the human body. It flourishes in the warm, moist environment of the GI and vaginal tracts.

A parasitic fungi, candida is present in everyone from the first few months of life and usually lives harmoniously in the body. What is destructive about this yeast overgrowth is how it changes from a harmless form to a dangerous invader. When this happens, it can affect nearly every organ in the body. In particular, it affects the GI tract, nervous system, genital and urinary tract, endocrine system, and immune system.

Candida Diet Notes

The classic candida diet permits dense protein foods, such as chicken and fish, and as many vegetables as you can eat. Some people can use whole grains, while others cannot. You should avoid caffeine and alcohol, and foods made with flour, such as breads, pastas, tortillas, cakes, and cookies. Eliminating the last two items and other foods made with sugar requires careful examination of food labels. Thousands of packaged foods contain sucrose, dextrose, glucose, fructose, corn syrup, maple syrup, honey, molasses, barley malt, rice syrup, or other forms of sugar.

You should also avoid foods with vinegar (mustard or mayonnaise); such fermented foods as cheese, sauerkraut, and soy sauce; and processed meats, especially hot dogs, sausages, and bacon. Try to drink only filtered or bottled water; tap water contains chlorine, which will further reduce the body's populations of friendly flora.

If you are a strict vegetarian, it is difficult to obtain enough complete protein without overloading on grains and beans. Eating a wide variety of vegetables at the same time can help counter this problem, as can supplements such as spirulina and chlorella. Books with recipes for the candida diet can be invaluable.

One reason yeast typically doesn't cause problems is the nearly three pounds of friendly bacteria in the intestines that help keep it in check by maintaining a balance of power between good bacteria and yeast. That is, until people upset this delicate balance with antibiotics, prednisone, hormones such as estrogen and progesterone, stress, diabetes, or by eating too much sugar and highly processed foods. If this overgrowth happens when your immune system is weakened, this once-harmless yeast can transform itself into an invasive fungal form.

This invader, called *mycelial form*, actually produces rootlike tentacles called *rhizoids*. These roots can penetrate through the lining of the GI tract, causing a painful condition briefly mentioned in the introduction. This is known as "leaky gut," which refers to increased intestinal permeability. When you have a leaky gut, partially digested food particles pass through the intestinal lining and directly enter the bloodstream. In addition, toxic waste produced by the candida also passes into the bloodstream. When this happens, food allergies can result, along with such symptoms as excessive bloating, gas, belching, heartburn, diarrhea, and constipation.

Candida symptoms

While yeast produces more than seventy-nine known toxins, probably the worst is acetaldehyde. When it enters the liver, it is converted into alcohol and contributes to a raft of harmful symptoms. They can include such ailments as fatigue, irritability, mental cloudiness, headaches, anxiety, or depression. In addition, yeast also depletes minerals, increases free radical formation, and disrupts enzymes needed to produce energy. If all this weren't bad enough, it produces other toxins that can make you feel miserable.

Given enough time, yeast can invade the bloodstream and affect all organs or tissues. As soon as it affects a particular organ, it produces symptoms. For instance, as candida or its toxic waste products damage the nervous system, you may experience fatigue, sleepiness, memory loss, attention deficit, insomnia, or other problems. Left unchecked, overgrowth can sweep through your entire body like an avalanche. Because yeast often affects the endocrine system, it eventually causes adrenal exhaustion and chronic fatigue, and possibly thyroid problems, or such skin issues as eczema, hives, psoriasis, and acne.

Candida Cure

One way to fight candida is with biotic silver (pure silver protein). This powerful natural antibiotic and antifungal solution kills and removes from the body all bacteria, viruses, and fungi within a short period of time. It has been classified by the Food and Drug Administration as a dietary mineral supplement. There are no side effects recorded in decades of use, and studies at the University of Toronto concluded that no toxicity, even in high dosages, results from its use.

Having sufficient pure silver protein in the body is like having a superior, second immune system. Long ago, when the earth was more fertile and the food supply more natural, silver in the soil would get absorbed into food. This in turn prevented infectious diseases, since no yeast, bacteria, or viruses can survive the presence of silver. However, due to extensive silver mining and silver inorganic farming methods, little remains in the soil. Research indicates that biotic silver protein has been used successfully in the treatment of more than 650 diseases. Among them are candida and yeast infections, as well as such ailments as allergies, athlete's foot, pneumonia, bladder infections, boils, infections, and cold sores. Biotic silver can even be given to infants and can be used during pregnancy.

Biotic silver is gold in color, tasteless, odorless, and does not upset the stomach. It is nontoxic, nonaddictive, nonaccumulative, and completely safe.

Once candida weakens the digestive system, it becomes increasingly difficult for your body to break down proteins into amino acids. When partially digested proteins called peptides are absorbed directly into the bloodstream, your immune system recognizes them as foreign invaders and forms antibodies to attack them. Often this immune reaction takes place in the lining of the small intestine, which causes more damage to the small intestines. A vicious cycle of destruction and allergic reactions can spiral out of control, with candida overgrowth robbing your body of vital nutrients.

Dietary Factors

Recovering from yeast overgrowth calls for key dietary changes for a period of time to fully restore your body's natural balance. How long depends on the severity of your yeast syndrome. The majority of those suffering from candida will need to stay on the diet for three months. Women with mild cases may only need to follow it for one to two months, while severe cases can mean six to twelve months.

The dietary causes are many, so try addressing the following:

A sweet tooth

The average American consumes about 150 pounds of sugar annually. Sugar-rich food is the single most important contributing factor, which is why you must avoid it for a season of time. This includes white sugar, brown sugar, syrups, honey, maltose, maple sugar, molasses, fructose, date sugar, and glucose, as well as the sugar in fruit juices and high-sugar vegetable juices (such as carrot juice). The herbal sweetener stevia is an excellent alternative to sugar, and Splenda is acceptable in moderation.

Milk products

Milk and milk products contain lactose, which encourages candida growth. Small amounts of butter are acceptable for less severe cases; other exceptions are lactose-free yogurt and kefir. Indeed, the latter are beneficial, since they contain good bacteria that helps to restore the bowel and can also act as a preventive agent. However, avoid yogurt and kefir containing sugar, fruit, or lactose, since these products will feed yeast.

Fruit

For the first three weeks of a yeast-free diet, omit fruits. After that, you may introduce less sweet kinds. Acceptable fruits include lemons, limes, apples, kiwi, blackberries, watermelon, grapefruit, raspberries, strawberries, and blueberries. Sweet fruits to avoid are dried fruits, bananas, cherries, grapes, peaches, plums, dried fruits, oranges, cantaloupe, honeydew, mangoes, and pineapple.

Dealing with carbs

Most people love carbs, especially breads and snack foods. While working to restore your body's balance, limiting refined carbohydrates is vital. Candida thrives on them, meaning they feed the overgrowth. Decreasing them slows the multiplication of yeast cells. This means avoiding such foods as white bread, pastas, muffins, pancakes, most breakfast cereals, potato chips, corn chips, and white crackers. In addition, decrease consumption of packaged and processed foods. Most are highly processed and, along with refined sugar, help yeast multiply.

However, some less-refined carbohydrates are desirable. Carbs that are safe include oats, buckwheat, millet bread, quinoa, brown rice, amaranth, spelt pasta, and spelt.

Whole wheat

Chapter 1 talked about the hazards of wheat consumption. With mild candida overgrowth, whole wheat may be fine. But if your case is in the moderate to severe range, you may be unable to tolerate whole wheat. If after eating whole-wheat products you develop bloating, belching, gas, mood changes, or other problems, you should avoid them for at least three months. Wheat is high in gluten, and many individuals with candida overgrowth are gluten-sensitive. For such individuals, eating whole-wheat products may worsen their candida. Oats also contain gluten, but in lower amounts than wheat. Again, if symptoms occur, avoid oats as well.

Other foods

There is a long list of foods to avoid, such as those with yeast or mold (all cheeses, most breads, and baked goods), condiments and sauces with yeast (mustard, ketchup, barbecue sauce) or those with vinegar (most salad dressings, mayonnaise), preserved and processed meats. Avoid most nuts—unless you purchase them in the shell and crack them open—as well as mushrooms, leftovers, alcohol, and allergy-causing foods such as eggs, dairy products, wheat, corn, yeast, chocolate, and citrus fruits.

Candida Management Breakthrough

With the advent of digestive enzymes, a new tool against candida has emerged. Since candida's cell wall is made largely of cellulose, cellulose enzymes break it down. As this occurs, the yeast dies. Cellulase enzymes do not harm the liver and are safe in every way. Further, because candida cannot change the structure of its cell wall, it cannot become immune to these enzymes. Finally, because the enzymes do not cause the yeast to release toxins, you will feel better almost immediately.

Candex is a natural yeast management by Pure Essence Labs (888-254-8000). Each capsule of Candex contains about 52,000 units of cellulose digesting activity. Most people respond best to about 200,000 CUs (Cellulase Units) of cellulase per day. Candex is the only product that is commonly available that provides these levels. It is available from health food stores, natural health practitioners, and physicians.

One caution, though: while some people say that after using Candex they have been able to reintroduce wider varieties of foods without incident, others report a rapid recurrence of discomfort when they do this.

Don't despair, though. There are many acceptable foods, starting with vegetables. Except for potatoes, sweet potatoes, and mushrooms, eating vegetables is one of the best ways to address candida overgrowth. Eat a minimum of three to five servings of vegetables a day. Although best eaten raw, you can lightly steam or stir-fry them as well, and create many varieties of vegetable soup.

Also, beans or legumes are high in protein and have about the same amount of calories as grains. High in fiber, this includes black beans, black-eyed peas, garbanzo beans, kidney beans, lentils, lima beans, pinto beans, red beans, soybeans, and split peas.

Meats, poultry, and fish do not feed candida. However, some animal feeds contain antibiotics, which remain in meat and can cause yeast to proliferate; thus, choose meat and poultry free of antibiotics, such as free-range beef and chicken. Eat fish at least three times a week, choosing fatty fish such as salmon, herring, mackerel, halibut, or sardines, which are high in omega-3 fatty acids.

You may also have lamb or veal, as well as two to three servings of eggs weekly.

Chapter 4

TREATING IBS

IRRITABLE BOWEL SYNDROME, or IBS, is also known as spastic colon or nervous stomach. It happens to be the most common gastrointestinal disorder, affecting one in five American adults—about thirty-five million people. Approximately twice as many women suffer from IBS as men, accounting for a whopping half of all visits to GI specialists and 10 percent of all family practitioner visits. It is a functional *gastrointestinal disorder*, which means that its symptoms cannot be explained by any anatomical, physiological, or biochemical abnormality. Since doctors can't identify with standard tests of the GI tract, IBS is diagnosed from its symptoms.

If you have IBS, your colon cannot always coordinate its function in a normal fashion; therefore, it spasms. It tends to be more sensitive to certain food triggers and various dietary factors. In addition, your colon can be where the body releases emotional responses through physical symptoms. This means your bowels can become a link between the spiritual conflict that you battle daily (the stress of a pressure-cooker world) and your physical body. So, if you are experiencing IBS, chances are good that your body has been in a battle, as well as your mind and spirit.

As mentioned, IBS is identified via its symptoms. You likely have IBS if you experience at least three of these six most common symptoms for more than three months.

Abdominal pain

This is the main symptom. It usually feels like a cramping pain, but may be either sharp or dull. It is commonly located in the left lower quadrant of the abdomen, below the belly button and to the left. However, the pain can be felt throughout the entire abdomen. This pain usually is relieved by having a bowel movement or by passing gas.

Irregular bowel function

You may experience episodes of irregular bowel function alternating with normal function. You may have constipation or diarrhea, or a combination of both.

19

Urgency to have a movement

Another symptom is the urgency to have a bowel movement, which can strike at any time, but usually at mealtimes or soon after. Not only is this urgency unpredictable, but it can prove very embarrassing.

Abdominal swelling

Another common symptom is abdominal swelling and bloating that generally occurs after eating. The pain and swelling usually subside with sleep.

Mucus in the stool

Mucus (without blood) in the stool is another symptom. Mucus is secreted by the lining of the colon and rectum, and it functions as a lubricant to ease stool passage. If you have IBS, your body may produce extra mucus, but it is not dangerous nor a sign of serious disease.

Incomplete emptying

Another common symptom is a feeling of incomplete emptying of the rectum. People suffering from IBS feel they have only had a partial bowel movement and strain in an attempt to pass more stool. This is hard on the anus and can lead to the development of hemorrhoids and eventually rectal prolapse (a condition where the lining of the rectum protrudes from the body).

Get diagnosed

If you have at least three of these six symptoms for more than three months without symptoms of a bowel disease, you probably have IBS. Nevertheless, only your doctor can make a final determination. If you are experiencing other painful symptoms, you may have an inflammatory bowel disease such as Crohn's disease or ulcerative colitis; therefore, it is vital to see your doctor for a correct diagnosis. Consult your physician in the event of these symptoms, which could indicate a more serious condition:

+ Blood in the stool
+ Sudden weight loss

+ Fevers
+ Waking up from sleep with bowel disturbances

The Basics of Bowel Movements

Those suffering from IBS should be aware that regularity and painful symptoms are closely related. A major cause of IBS is an inconsistency in the speed at which your stools pass through your GI tract. If they pass too fast, you will develop diarrhea. But if they pass too slowly, you will become constipated— passing a hard, small stool or having fewer than three bowel movements per week. When the stool is small and hard from constipation, then the colon has to work much harder to eliminate it. This built-up pressure can lead to spasms and cramps that create a great deal of pain.

If you do not drink enough water and eat enough fiber, or if you neglect natural urges to go to the bathroom, you are likely to become constipated. However, it has many other causes, such as taking prescription medications (narcotics, pain medications, hypertension aids), antacids, antihistamines, and even iron tablets. A lack of exercise can also contribute to constipation.

Causes

The roots of IBS are linked to many factors of physical, mental, and emotional depletion, including fatigue, chronic stress, long-term emotional turmoil, and much more. Resolving the situation may call for more than simple adjustments in your diet. A consultation with your primary care physician and any experts he or she recommends may be in order.

Among the physical situations that can be at fault are intestinal assaults such as food poisoning. An infection of the intestinal tract known as *gastroenteritis* can cause IBS. Salmonella, a species of pathogenic bacteria, is often the culprit. Infections are usually caused by improperly preparing and cooking chicken, eggs, and other meats.

Some other physical causes include the following:

+ Parasites and viruses

    Intestinal parasites are protozoa or worms that live off a host (you) and damage the GI tract. Infections are common in the United States, where researchers have identified more than 130 species of intestinal parasites. Fortunately, the IBS that develops after parasitic gastroenteritis usually only lasts for a few weeks.

+ Lactose intolerance

This is the inability to properly digest milk and milk products. Its symptoms are similar to those of IBS, though classified as a separate condition, and may include diarrhea, bloating, gas, and abdominal cramps. This intolerance affects 20 percent of Caucasians, 75 percent of African Americans, 80 percent of Asian Americans, and 50 percent of Hispanics.

+ Antibiotics

While antibiotics are modern wonders that have helped many, extended use can lead to IBS. So can even short-term use of powerful antibiotics. Despite aggressively attacking infections, they can also wreak havoc on intestinal flora and affect the delicate balance of good bacteria. Plus, antibiotics taken to cure infections can cause a colon infection; overuse can lead to bacterial overgrowth in the small intestine.

+ Candida and leaky gut syndrome (refer to chapter 3)

Since a poor diet is a major contributor to IBS, addressing your food intake will certainly help you move toward a cure. So will such steps as getting adequate rest, de-stressing your life, and paying attention to prayer and your spiritual life. Mind, body, and spirit are interrelated, so what affects one affects the others.

Some commonsense steps toward addressing nutritional balance to attack IBS include identifying food triggers—those foods that make your symptoms worse. If you exhibit symptoms, avoid such things as hot sauce, barbecue sauce, salsa, hot peppers, chili powder, and caffeine (coffee, tea, and most sodas).

For diabetics or dieters, sugar-free foods tend to trigger IBS too. Many times the reason for this is the sorbitol, an artificial sweetener found in sugar-free gums, diet chocolates, sugar-free candies, and some apple products (juice, cider, canned fruits). Study the labels of all fruit and sugar-free products before purchasing them to see if they contain sorbitol.

Fructose is a common IBS food trigger, often causing bloating, gas, and diarrhea. Foods you should avoid are dried fruits, fruit juices, raisins, figs, dates, soft drinks, fruit juices, honey, and most candies.

Other foods to avoid are gassy foods (such as legumes, beans, brussels sprouts, cabbage, broccoli), wheat products, fats (fried foods, butter, mayonnaise, fatty cuts of meat, and other high-fat foods), the fat substitute Olestra, alcohol, and excessive fiber.

BETTER EATING HABITS

Most people with IBS have poor eating patterns that make their condition much worse. Here is a description of the eating habits of a typical IBS patient—see if you are reflected in this scenario: For breakfast, the IBS sufferer grabs a convenience store doughnut and washes it down with hot coffee while fighting rush hour traffic. Then the person skips lunch, but grabs cookies on a break and washes them down with a diet soda. Feeling too stressed to cook dinner, she picks up the evening meal at the drive-through window.

Sound familiar? It reflects the pattern of many IBS sufferers who compound their poor nutritional habits by eating under stressful circumstances, or when tense and angry. This is terrible for your GI tract. So is eating too fast, reflected by lunches and dinners that resemble a track meet. God created food for you to savor, not chew so quickly and inadequately you have to wash it down with a beverage. To ensure proper digestion means chewing every bite of food at least twenty to thirty times. You may have to make a real effort to slow down at meal times, since American culture not only eats too fast, but often skips the leisurely social interaction of family dinners.

Natural Remedies for IBS

If you are among the thirty-five million adults suffering from Irritable Bowel Syndrome, here are a couple methods of dealing with IBS. Calm Colon is an effective irritable bowel syndrome formula, clinically proven for internal bowel support. Calm Colon was proven effective in double-blind placebo-controlled clinical trials. Treatment includes taking one capsule, three times daily. (You can order Calm Colon by calling 800-669-2256.)

IBS can also be controlled with two herbs:

- Peppermint relaxes the smooth muscle surrounding the large intestine, curbing spasms. During flare-ups take one or two enteric-coated peppermint oil capsules three times daily between meals.

- St. John's wort acts as a mild tranquilizer and antidepressant, thereby relieving emotional stress. Take one capsule two times daily with meals.[1]

Skipping meals is another bad habit you need to avoid, since it often results in consuming massive quantities of food late in the evening. Never skip meals, and always allow about three to four hours between meals, as well as between your last meal and bedtime. Give your GI tract a chance to digest your food. In addition, don't overeat. Decide before meals how much to eat, and skip seconds and sugary deserts. Practice learning to stop eating as soon as you are satisfied so you don't stuff yourself. Finally, don't be a "junk food junkie." Avoid fast foods, chips, french fries, pastries, doughnuts, cookies, pies, fried foods, and candy bars.

Keeping these eating guidelines in mind every day will take you a long way in overcoming painful IBS symptoms. How you eat and what you eat are major keys to winning this battle.

Chapter 5

FIBER AND REGULARITY

WHEN IT COMES to achieving and maintaining a healthy gut, eating more fiber should be at the top of your list. Why? Because a lack of fiber can lead to a clogged colon. So can such factors as dehydration (lack of water), a lack of walking and exercise, lack of enzymes in your food, and prescriptions and over-the-counter drugs. If you are not having a bowel movement at least once a day, then technically you are constipated and your bowels are sluggish. And, if you do not experience at least three bowel movements daily, then you have a clogged colon. (Many Americans have only three bowel movements a week.) During autopsies, pathologists have discovered up to thirty pounds of non-digested, putrefied fecal matter in human colons. Such clogging contributed to these people's deaths.

Along with nuts, seeds, beans, and essential fatty acids, fiber is one of the "living" nutrients recommended by health experts to keep your gut in good condition. Fresh fruits and vegetables contain more than just fiber; they are rich in the enzymes your system needs to digest your food, vitamins, and minerals. Fruits and vegetables also have antioxidant benefits and help to keep your arteries clear and free of clogs.

Fantastic Fiber

If you need to get more fiber into your diet, PGX—which is short for PolyGlycoPlex—is one way. PGX is a unique blend of highly viscous fibers that act synergistically to create a much higher level of viscosity than the individual fibers alone. PGX absorbs hundreds of times its weight in water over one to two hours and expands in the digestive tract, creating a thick gelatinous material. It creates a feeling of fullness, stabilizes blood sugar and insulin levels, and stabilizes appetite hormones.

PGX lowers blood sugar after eating by about 20 percent and lowers insulin secretion by about 40 percent. Researchers

have found that higher doses of PGX can decrease appetite
significantly. PGX works similarly to gastric banding and has
fewer gastrointestinal side effects than other viscous dietary
fibers. However, start slowly, or you may develop gas. Try two
or three capsules with sixteen ounces of water before every
meal and gradually increase the dose if needed.

Fiber is a form of carbohydrate not absorbed by the body. However,
fiber slows down the rate of absorption of other carbohydrates. Thus,
the higher the fiber content of the carbohydrate or starch, the more
slowly the body will absorb it as it enters the bloodstream. In addition to
their high fiber content, most fruits and vegetables have a low glycemic
index (GI) rating. This refers to a ranking of carbohydrates on a scale
from 0 to 100 according to how much they raise blood sugar levels after
eating. The only fruits with a high glycemic index are bananas, raisins,
dates, and other dried fruits. The only vegetables with a high GI rating
are potatoes, carrots, corn, and beets.

Whole fruits and vegetables have insoluble and soluble fiber. Both
types of fiber are important for colon health, while soluble fiber is excellent for the digestive tract. It also helps to lower blood cholesterol, stabilize blood sugar, and improve good bowel bacteria. Fiber not only
improves gut health, but it also aids in weight loss because fiber slows the
passage of food through the digestive tract. This decreases the absorption of sugars and starches into the stomach, and expands and fills up the
stomach, which turns down the appetite. However, the standard diet followed by millions in the United States falls well short of recommended
fiber intake. The American Heart Association and the National Cancer
Institute recommend thirty grams or more of fiber each day, but the
average American only consumes between twelve and seventeen grams.[1]

High-Fiber Foods

If you need to get more fiber to improve the condition of your
gut, here is a quick reference guide of foods high in fiber:

- Oatmeal
- Plums
- Almonds
- Corn (cooked)
- Apple with skin
- Carrots (cooked)
- Brown rice
- Pinto beans
- Nectarine
- Dates

- Banana
- Brazil nuts
- Pineapple (raw)
- Raisins
- Spinach (cooked)
- Papaya
- Blueberries
- Honeydew

- Whole cranberries
- Lima beans
- Bran
- Dried prunes
- Seeds and nuts
- Raw vegetables
- Whole-grain cereals
- Potato with skin (baked)
- Brussels sprouts (cooked)

If your fiber intake is below average, you may not realize all the benefits you are missing. Soluble fiber lowers the blood sugar, slowing down digestion and the absorption of sugars and carbohydrates. This allows for a more gradual rise in blood sugar, which lowers the glycemic index of the foods you eat and helps to improve blood sugar levels. Plus, a little fiber goes a long way. One study found that consuming an extra fourteen grams of soluble fiber each day for only two days was associated with a 10 percent decrease in caloric intake.[2] Add a few pieces of fruit and several servings of vegetables to your daily diet, and you can obtain that extra fourteen grams.

There are many sources of fiber. In addition to fruits and vegetables, there are many grains. Some examples:

- Wheat fiber from bran-type cereals; it has also been proven successful in preventing certain types of cancer. Try to get a half-cup daily.
- Oat fiber (oat bran) may lower blood-fat levels (cholesterol). Consider including one-third cup of an oat bran cereal daily (may be mixed with wheat bran).
- Beans and peas. You should eat these regularly, preferably three times weekly. While canned beans, peas, and corn are all good sources of fiber, vitamins, and minerals, they are not

as nutritious as fresh—use them for convenience only when necessary.

Keep It Clean

Your fiber intake has a major role in proper elimination. Poor elimination contributes to most adverse health conditions. Old, impacted waste material often reabsorbs into the body and nearby organs and sets the stage for diseases, viruses, parasites, and candida. While the causes of constipation are varied, a leading culprit is a low-fiber diet. Others include stress, a poor diet with too much sugar, processed foods, prescription drugs, and a lack of exercise.

Fiber guards against internal toxicity that can also harm your health. A leading cause of this toxicity is a poor diet with a lack of live foods (fresh fruit and vegetables), a lack of proper enzyme activity, constipation, and a lack of water to flush toxins and speed up the digestive and eliminative process. A diet high in fiber and low in animal fat can act as a personal insurance policy against internal toxicity. In other words, go heavy on the fresh fruits and vegetables while skipping the cheeseburgers, french fries, and cream-filled doughnuts. These dietary considerations will have a two-pronged effect:

1. It will prevent improper elimination.

2. It will prevent or help to heal the diseases elimination problems cause.

Unreleased waste can be a breeding ground for the parasitic infections mentioned in the previous chapter. Intestinal parasites feed on fermented, rancid, and overaccumulated amounts of food in the intestinal tract. This can lead to lowered immunity, tissue degeneration, poor circulation, and sluggish organ and glandular function. There are obvious symptoms of an unhealthy digestive tract: poor digestion, bad breath, lower backache, fatigue, and gas, to name a few.

Pay attention to stress levels too, since stress also hinders proper digestion, absorption, and elimination. Lowering stress is part of adopting a healthy lifestyle that results in good colon health. If you aren't already, you should initiate a walking program to stimulate circulation. (Consult your doctor when starting any new exercise routine.) Exercise stimulates the circulatory and lymphatic systems, and can help release stress. It raises metabolic efficiency and enhances the body's natural cleansing ability.

If your body feels sluggish, or you know you have IBS or other problems with elimination, consider colonic irrigation given by a colonic therapist.

As for food habits, in addition to avoiding sugar, animal fats, fried foods, and dairy foods, you should drink six to eight glasses of water daily. (More about that in chapter 12.) Add fiber foods to improve transit time for food moving through in your gut, which should be ten to twelve hours.

Bad Bread

You need more fiber in your diet, but don't expect to get it from eating white bread or the gooey yeast rolls that are popular in so many restaurants. Take a look at how most American bread is made. First the outer shell of the grain of wheat is removed. This is the bran or the fiber portion of the grain. The germ of the wheat is then removed; the germ contains the essential fats and vitamin E. These are removed to affect the shelf life of the bread. What is left over is the endosperm, which is the starch, which is then ground into a fine powder. Since this granular powder is not white, it is bleached.

With both the bran and wheat germ gone, after this bleaching process few vitamins remain. So bakers add back man-made vitamins, along with sugar, salt, partially hydrogenated fats, and preservatives. Because it contains no fiber, white bread is very constipating. Since it is highly processed, the body rapidly breaks it down into sugars at the time of consumption. This causes the body to secrete high amounts of insulin, putting a strain on the pancreas and programming the body to store fat. This is hardly the kind of bread that contributes to healthy life.

Diverticulosis

Diverticulosis is a condition in which excess pressure builds up inside the colon, usually caused by constipation or hard stool. This promotes the development of multiple small pouches, called diverticula, in the wall of the large intestine. The more serious disease of diverticulitis occurs when the small pouches become infected and inflamed. This common condition affects about 40 percent of Americans over the age of fifty.[3] The best way to prevent this painful and problematic illness is to soften the stools and keep them regular by adding fiber to the diet. Eating oatmeal or Kellogg's All-Bran Buds cereal each morning is a good way to accomplish this, as it contains two different fibers and has been shown effective in maintaining stool regularity.

A lack of fiber in the diet can both cause and lead to other problems. A diet with too many refined foods and a lack of fiber leads to a weakened colon wall. Plus, a diet low in fiber leads to chronic constipation and gas, which worsens the condition. Such painful symptoms can create emotional stress, a cause of colon spasms. A poor diet that leads to obesity, among other things, can result in a prolapsed colon structure. Symptoms can include abdominal cramping and pain, distention, diarrhea, and rectal bleeding.

In addition to adding oatmeal and cereals such as Bran Buds for breakfast to address diverticulosis, you can also try eating yogurt and lean protein (tofu, seafood, beans, brown rice); eliminating dairy, fatty, fried, and sugary foods; and avoiding nuts and seeds.

Supplements that will help include B-complex vitamins, magnesium chloride liquid to reduce spasms, wild yam capsules, evening primrose oil, L-glutamine, echinacea-goldenseal capsules, theanine to reduce stress, a daily green drink such as Kyo-Green, and Bio-K Liquid Acidophilus during acute phase, followed by daily Kyo-Dophilus capsules when it lessens.

Chapter 6

INFLAMMATION

ALTHOUGH RESEARCH IS continuing, inflammation is often linked with heart attacks, strokes, and other problems stemming from clogged arteries. However, inflammation also represents a serious problem when it comes to gut health. Take the various gastric diseases that affect Americans' gastrointestinal tracts. Gastric disease is characterized by inflammation of the stomach and intestinal tract. It also involves the leaking of stomach acid back into the lower esophagus and acid coming up into the throat.

Symptoms include excess gas, belching, bloating, and heartburn, as well as irritable bowels, sharp abdominal pains, chest pains, and shortness of breath. After eating, sufferers may experience such problems as poor digestion, hiccups, pressure behind the breastbone, diarrhea, or difficulty swallowing.

Gastritis, gastroenteritis, and gastric ulcers are ulcerative disorders of the GI tract. In addition, ulcers linked to lifestyles are common. Stress, poor diet, and long-term use of anti-inflammatory medications (NSAIDs) cause ulcers and gastrointestinal bleeding. A chronic sinus condition with postnasal drip also contributes to these diseases. With all of the stress, poor dietary habits, improper food combinations, and enzyme-deficient foods to which people are exposed, it is no wonder that gastric disease has risen sharply in the past two decades.

Dealing with diseases of the GI tract starts with making small, seemingly innocuous changes. For example, do not eat when emotionally upset, and do not lie down immediately after eating. Do not smoke. If you are overweight, plan to lose weight. Practice deep-breathing exercises to promote relaxation. Deep breathing will bring noticeable improvements to physical workouts, curtail problems with fatigue, and enhance sleep patterns. As part of your lifestyle change, eat only small meals, chew all food thoroughly, and avoid eating late at night. During flare-ups, eat raw and lightly steamed vegetables. Avoid fried and spicy foods.

Anti-Inflammatory Diet

To reduce inflammation in your body, try avoiding all gluten (wheat, barley, rye, spelt). This includes all products made with these grains, including bread, pasta, crackers, bagels, pretzels, and most cereals. Go to www.celiacsociety.com for a comprehensive list of gluten-free foods. Also avoid corn products except for corn on the cob. Choose non-genetically modified (non-GMO) varieties.

In addition to changing the way you eat, consider weekly chiropractic treatments or massage therapy until you see improvement in your condition. Realize that antacids can cause more problems in the long term, since they may cause kidney stones and contribute to high blood pressure. In addition, those that contain aluminum may raise the risk of aluminum toxicity. Avoid NSAID medications, especially if you have an ulcer.

People with hiatal hernias should avoid chocolate, alcohol, red meat, coffee, and carbonated beverages. Add therapeutic juices, such as freshly made carrot juice, carrot-cabbage juice, and carrot-papaya juice. Healthy teas include chamomile and Pau d'Arco. Supplements that will help include MSM, Gastro and Purify (from Enzymedica), magnesium, glutamine powder (500 mg three times daily), Ester-C (3,000 mg daily), Kyo-Dophilus before meals, and a daily green drink (such as Kyo-Green).

Other Inflammatory Problems

Colitis

Colitis is an inflammation of the large intestine, accompanied by diarrhea, constipation, and cramping. It may be caused by emotional stress, depression and anxiety, lack of fiber, food allergies, candida, a vitamin K deficiency, overuse of antibiotics, and excess sugar and refined foods in the diet. Symptoms include pain, gas, bloody diarrhea, ulcers in the colon lining, and hard stools.

Most colitis sufferers are between the ages of twenty and forty, with stressful occupations or lifestyles. Females are slightly more prone to colitis than males.[1] Most cases are related to food allergies, which in turn cause an inflamed colon. Cheese, corn, wheat, and eggs are the most common colitis triggers. Diet change is imperative in relieving and healing colitis.

Addressing this condition starts with cleaning up your diet. Add oatmeal, brown rice, steamed veggies, green salads, fresh fruits—especially apples—and yogurt to your daily diet. Eat smaller meals, which will make it easier for you to digest and assimilate your food. Avoid coffee and other foods containing caffeine, nuts, dairy products, and citrus foods. In addition, cut out sugar, wheat, and spicy foods. Drink at least six to eight glasses of water daily, making one of those glasses a green drink.

Supplements that will help deal with colitis include milk thistle extract for liver health, and Bio-K probiotic culture liquid for intestinal rebalancing and rebuilding. Take glucosamine sulfate (500 mg) daily for mucous membrane rebuilding, royal jelly for adrenal gland health, and Siberian ginseng to fortify the body during times of stress. For cramping, try cramp bark capsules. Before bed, have a cup of chamomile tea sweetened with stevia. Or, calm the body with kava, valerian, or passionflower tea.

Inflammation Fighters

Ginger is a spice that will help improve your gut health in several ways. It contains a substance that stimulates gastric enzymes, which can boost metabolism. The better your metabolism, the more calories you will burn. In addition to its anti-inflammatory qualities, ginger has been shown to improve gastric motility, the spontaneous peristaltic movements of the stomach that aid in moving food through the digestive system. This means less bloating and constipation. It has also been found to lower cholesterol. Also, ginger is the top vegan source of zinc, which boosts your immune system. Top that off with the fact that it tastes delicious in juice recipes, and you have a super spice.

Chili peppers contain a substance known as capsaicin, which gives peppers their spicy taste. Capsaicin inhibits substance P, a neuropeptide associated with inflammation. The hotter the chili pepper, the more capsaicin. The hottest varieties are habanero, followed by Scotch bonnet; the mildest are Spanish pimentos, Anaheim, and Hungarian cherry peppers.

Capsaicin has been studied as a treatment for arthritis, psoriasis, and diabetic neuropathy. When animals were injected with a substance that causes inflammatory arthritis and were fed capsaicin in their diet, they had delayed onset of arthritis and reduced inflammation.[2]

Crohn's disease

Also known as regional enteritis, this is a chronic inflammation of the digestive tract accompanied by painful ulcers. These ulcers may form in one or more sections of the gastrointestinal tract. Other symptoms include diarrhea, abdominal pain, low-grade fever, weight loss, depression, anemia, wheat sensitivity, gas, inflammation, and soreness. Even worse, the immune system function declines due to malnutrition. This painful autoimmune disease affects over two million Americans today, and the numbers are rising.[3] This is mostly because so many people consistently eat diets low in fiber and high in refined sugar. Other contributors are food allergies, yeast overgrowth, and emotional stress.

Crohn's sufferers should gradually increase fiber intake until they are eating a substantially high-fiber diet—except during flare-ups. Drink eight to ten glasses of spring water daily. Consume fresh juices and vegetables daily (grape, carrot, apple, and pineapple are especially therapeutic). Avoid red and fatty meats, dairy products, and fried foods. Eliminate seeds, popcorn, and nuts.

Lifestyle changes will help, starting with reducing stress factors and getting regular massages. Practice deep breathing. Eat early in the day, reducing the size of your meals but eating more often. Supplements that will help include magnesium (400-800 mg daily); Bio-K Liquid Acidophilus during flare-ups, then Kyo-Dophilus capsules; glutamine (500 mg); vitamin C; royal jelly; quercetin; Kyolic Garlic capsules (six daily); green tea; flax oil; daily green drink; and peppermint tea.

Chapter 7

THE AUTOIMMUNE COLLECTION

IN THE PREVIOUS chapter we looked at the problems inflammation causes in your gut. However, the modern Western diet leads to many other diseases, which is why paying attention to gut health can produce additional benefits for your body. Other problems related to inflammation range from allergies and weight gain to autoimmune disorders, Alzheimer's disease, cardiovascular disease, cancer, diabetes, arthritis, asthma, and prostate problems.

Here's why. There are several deadly by-products of a high-fat, high-processed, high-sugar, high-grain (wheat and corn), and high-sodium diet. This type of diet throws off the balance in the body between inflammatory and anti-inflammatory chemicals called prostaglandins. Normally, inflammation is a good thing, working to repair an injury or fight off infection. It also puts the immune system on high alert to attack invading bacteria or viruses. In case of an injury, it rushes white blood cells to the cut, scrape, sprain, or broken bone; thus, the body removes damaged cells, splints the injury, or attacks infections. This is the good side of inflammation and an important function of the immune system's small agents.

When your body faces an emergency, it goes through a complicated process to create more pro-inflammatory prostaglandins than anti-inflammatory ones. The immune system responds to the alarm. When the crisis ends, the balance swings in the anti-inflammatory direction and eventually balances out again. In a simplified sense, prostaglandins are produced from the foods we eat in an ongoing cycle. Each of the foods we eat has either a pro-inflammatory tendency or an anti-inflammatory one. Fatty acids are at the center of this. Omega-6 fatty acids are "friendly" to the creation of pro-inflammatory prostaglandins, while omega-3 fatty acids are "friendly" to the creation of anti-inflammatory prostaglandins.

A more natural diet emphasizing fruits, vegetables, nuts, and other natural substances will have a balance of pro- and anti-inflammatory-friendly foods. But the typical Western diet produces more pro-inflammatory prostaglandins. Experts say that since 1940, the standard American diet has doubled the amount of omega-6 fatty acids consumed by shifting away from fruits and vegetables to grain-based foods and oils. Most people eat about twenty times more omega-6s than anti-inflammatory omega-3s. Most animals are grain fed, so most meats, eggs, and dairy products are higher in omega-6s than they were a century ago. Most fish are now farm raised, eating a diet of cereal grains, so even much of the fish Americans consume represent higher sources of omega-6s than before.

Fish: Watch What Kind

Eating more fish is one way to keep inflammation problems in your body at bay. However, although fish is generally good for this and a healthy protein choice, some contain high levels of mercury. The following lists will help you determine which fish to eat more liberally and which to avoid.[1]

Fish with the least amounts of mercury include anchovies, catfish, crab, flounder, haddock (Atlantic), herring, salmon (fresh or canned), sardines, shrimp, sole, tilapia, trout (freshwater), and whitefish.

Fish with moderate amounts of mercury should be limited to a maximum of six servings per month. They include bass (striped or black), halibut (Atlantic or Pacific), lobster, mahi-mahi, monkfish, snapper, and tuna (canned, chunk light).

With fish high in mercury, you should limit consumption to no more than three servings per month: bluefish, grouper, mackerel (Spanish and Gulf), sea bass (Chilean), tuna (canned albacore or yellowfin). The fish that are highest in mercury and should be avoided are mackerel (king), marlin, orange roughy, and shark.

Chronic Problems

Noting all of this, it is easy to see why diseases caused by chronic systemic inflammation have grown to such proportions. Furthermore, essential fatty acids (EFAs) such as omega-3 and omega-6 cannot be manufactured in the body; they must be consumed through diet or supplements. With the high omega-6 content of the traditional Western diet, over time the natural, ongoing creation of prostaglandins has tipped toward systemic inflammation.

Despite the absence of an actual emergency, this imbalance sets off alarms calling for chronic or long-term inflammation. The immune system will respond accordingly. However, with no actual threat present, the immune system will start attacking things it normally wouldn't. This immune hypersensitivity is what leads to the various problems and diseases mentioned at the beginning of this chapter.

Many of these happen because as the immune system stays on high alert longer than it should, its agents begin to fatigue and make bad decisions, possibly leading to autoimmune disease or not destroying mutated cells. This causes many problems and frequently leads to cancer formation, often giving cancer a foothold it won't easily relinquish.

To ward off such situations, strive to consume more beneficial omega-3 fatty acids. Among healthy omega-3 foods for your diet are flaxseeds and flaxseed oil, chia seeds, salba seeds, hemp seeds, fish (wild salmon, sardines, tongol tuna, herring, and cod), and fish oil. Even if you are following a healthy diet regimen, within that framework you should also look at the pro-inflammatory or anti-inflammatory qualities of the foods you eat. If you are having problems with allergies, joint pains, muscle aches, or the like, eating more anti-inflammatory foods can help tip your balance back in the right direction.

One way to check your degree of inflammation is to have a C-reactive protein blood test. C-reactive protein is a promoter of inflammation and also a blood marker of systemic inflammation. Once you reach forty years of age, annual CRP testing is a great idea for checking the anti-inflammatory effectiveness of your diet. Men should aim for a CRP less than 1.0, while women should aim for a CRP less than 1.5.

Self-Directed Attacks

When the body's immune system goes haywire, instead of attacking a foreign invader, it attacks the body itself. For example, in multiple sclerosis the body literally attacks the myelin sheath that lines the nerve endings. In inflammatory bowel disease, including Crohn's disease and ileitis, the body attacks its own lower digestive tract. Interestingly, autoimmune diseases are much more common among women than they are among men, possibly due to a hormonal relationship that researchers are still studying.

To gain an understanding of what happens when things go awry in your immune system, consider how it was designed to function. The human body contains a vast array of various kinds of cells—white blood cells, lymphocytes, T-cells, and natural killer cells—all intended to ward off any invasions of the body, especially those that would cause a catastrophic illness. Scientists call certain kinds of cells "natural killer cells" because their job is to hunt down and kill these foreign, disease-causing invaders. One of these types of killer cells is called a *macrophage*, meaning "big eater." Much like Pac-Man in the old video game, the macrophage is designed to kill any foreign substances entering the body.

Royal Jelly

Taking a couple of teaspoons of royal jelly each day provides a blessing for the body against immune suppression, as well as asthma, liver disease, and skin disorders. This is because royal jelly is rich in vitamins, minerals, enzymes, and hormones. In addition, it possesses antibiotic and antibacterial properties.

It is interesting to note that royal jelly naturally contains a high concentration of pantothenic acid. Pantothenic acid is a B vitamin that plays a role in the production of adrenal hormones. Known as an antistress vitamin, pantothenic acid is helpful in alleviating anxiety and depression by fortifying the adrenal glands. In addition, pantothenic acid is needed to produce our own natural pain relievers, including cortisol. This is very important, because pain often goes hand in hand with emotional depletion—and depleted emotions can contribute to gut diseases.

Proper functioning of the T-cells is crucial because they act as the "commanders of the army," directing the macrophages into battle. Every time your body wards off germ warfare such as a cold, thank God for designing your immune system to turn away plagues from your dwelling (to paraphrase Psalm 91:10).

So many times, when people think of diseases of the immune system, they jump to the conclusion that these diseases occur when the immune system has somehow been compromised or knocked out altogether. A classic example would be the AIDS virus, which results in the immune system becoming deficient and underactive, leaving the person vulnerable to any number of contagious and deadly diseases. AIDS itself is not what kills a person; the diseases to which the person is helplessly exposed due to an underactive immune system strike the fatal blow.

An underactive immune system is not the only way the body becomes compromised. Serious problems can also occur if the body's immune system becomes *overactive*. If it reaches the point where the body's defenses begin to *attack itself*, a whole new category of illnesses—the autoimmune disorders mentioned at the start of this chapter—is the result.

Missing the Root Cause

Traditional medicine typically attempts to treat these diseases individually by coming up with such things as a new antibiotic to combat viruses or new nasal sprays to alleviate allergy symptoms. While they have their place, none deals with the root cause: an immune system that is out of balance. How many times have you been treated for a recurring virus with another round of antibiotics? Antibiotics can be harmful to our bodies because they kill not only the bad bacteria but also the good intestinal bacteria that promote healthy immune system function.

The times in which we live are dangerous. The threat of bioterrorism has become increasingly real. The fear used to be that some diseases, such as smallpox, might accidentally reappear. Now the fear is that they will be released on the world intentionally. In addition, new strains of viruses that have never before been reported in the United States are now on the rise, such as the Ebola virus and the West Nile virus, two of the most deadly.

In the development of "cures" for these diseases, traditional medicine inadvertently can create as much harm as good. For years the drug methicillin was used to kill off the deadly *Staphylococcus* bacteria, but now much of these bacteria have become resistant to the drug.

The key is to find balance. Proper nutrition can help restore the immune system to a healthy balance, in which it responds correctly to dangerous situations but lets harmless particles through without a fuss.

Chapter 8

SUPERFOODS FOR THE GUT

THERE IS A basic reason your gut needs nutritious foods that balance good and bad bacteria and aid digestion. Without effective bacterial function, the gut wall is vulnerable to invasion by opportunistic flora such as candida and toxins. Chronic inflammation can result, along with injury to the digestive system. Another function of gut bacteria is to provide energy and nourishment for the cells lining the gut wall. If abnormal gut flora takes over and harms gut wall cells, it leaves them incapable of digesting and absorbing nutrients. With normal, balanced gut flora working in concert with well-nourished gut wall cells, your body can better digest proteins, ferment carbohydrates, and proceed with normal breakdown of lipids and fiber.

Any damage to gut flora can result in reduced flow of nutrients through the gut wall into the bloodstream. Inflammation from numerous causes can damage gut flora. This leads to the previously mentioned leaky gut, where the gut wall becomes pervious due to faulty barrier function. The result is that any food that is not digested completely or any toxin that gains access into the bloodstream can cause damage to the nervous system, immune system, or other bodily systems.

Essentially the intestinal tract is a hidden ecosystem, or microbiome. This microbiome consists of over one hundred trillion microorganisms; your body consists of many trillions of cells. You live in a symbiotic, macro/micro relationship (one ecosystem), where one party cannot live without the other. In this ecosystem, your challenge is to ingest enough essential, beneficial flora. If the beneficial flora is reduced in number or becomes dysfunctional, what is known as opportunistic flora takes over, creating numerous health problems.

When it comes to foods that provide good bacteria for your gut, few things are as good as yogurt. It contains living organisms that help with the balance of good and bad bacteria, as well as digestion. Yogurt has

41

other benefits. Its high calcium content can inhibit the division of breast cancer cells, and its calcium and vitamin D are good for bone health.

Of course, since it is a dairy product and contains yeast, people suffering from lactose intolerance or yeast infections must take precautions. Nor can you eat all the yogurt you like, since dairy should be limited to four to six ounces every three days. Be careful to stay away from commercial products with added sugar and flavoring. One alternative is Greek yogurt, which is simply yogurt that has been strained to remove the whey. Greek yogurt contains less sugar, less sodium, and twice the amount of protein. The best is fat free and organic, and without added fruit. (Avoid frozen yogurt too.)

Other Gut Boosters

Garlic

Garlic is a prebiotic that enhances your gut microbiome, stimulates the immune system function, and has heart-protective effects. Plus, there are thirty different cancer-fighting compounds in garlic. It also helps fight infection; detoxifies the body; enhances immunity; lowers blood fats; assists in fighting yeast infections; and can help combat asthma, cancer, sinusitis, circulatory problems, and heart conditions.

A person with an unhealthy gut who is also battling overweight conditions should remember garlic's value as an appetite suppressant. The strong odor of garlic stimulates the brain's satiety center, thereby reducing feelings of hunger. It also increases the brain's sensitivity to leptin, a hormone produced by fat cells that regulates appetite. Further, garlic stimulates the nervous system to release hormones such as adrenaline, which speeds up metabolic rate. This means a greater ability to burn calories.

Garlic is used for many different reasons; it affects multiple body systems. It has been found to alter cholesterol levels and enhance the cardiovascular system. Studies indicate that garlic tends to be a mood elevator too, with regular users reporting less irritability, fatigue, and anxiety. In addition to helping your gut, garlic is a great food to eat during cold and flu season, since it can fight viruses and bacteria. If you can't handle the breath odors of fresh garlic, try a daily capsule form. (Check the label to be certain a capsule is the equivalent of one clove of fresh garlic.) Garlic bulb extract should be taken at a dose of 120 milligrams per day. Also, you can buy odorless garlic, such as Kyolic, made by Wakunaga.

Green superfoods

One of the best tools for building health is found in the class of foods called "green superfoods." They are supercharged with nutrition that boosts the immune system and improves digestion and elimination. Eating them is like receiving a small transfusion to enhance immunity and promote energy and well-being. These superfoods are purposely grown and harvested to maximize and ensure high vitamin, mineral, and amino acid concentrations. One of the best green foods for your gut is barley grass, which helps with inflammatory conditions of the stomach and digestive system. It contains vitamins, minerals, proteins, enzymes, chlorophyll, and more calcium than cow's milk, as well as vitamins C and B_{12}. Barley grass also helps combat inflammatory conditions of the stomach and digestive system.

The following are other superfoods available in most health food stores:

+ Blue and blue-green algae are the most potent sources of beta-carotene available. They are called the perfect superfoods because they are brimming with superior quality proteins, fiber, vitamins, minerals, and enzymes.

+ Spirulina is extremely high in protein and rich in B vitamins, amino acids, beta-carotene, and essential fatty acids. Easy to digest, it boosts energy quickly and sustains it for long periods of time.

+ Wheatgrass has been used around the world for many serious diseases to rebuild, cleanse, and strengthen the body because of its incredible nutritional value.

+ Kyo-Green by Wakunaga of America contains barley, wheatgrass, chlorella, and kelp. This is a potent formula that helps cleanse the bloodstream, detoxify the system, and supply the body with minerals, enzymes, and many important nutrients. This provides energy for enhanced daily performance.

These high-chlorophyll foods are very nutrient dense and are excellent sources of essential amino acids, vitamins, minerals, essential fatty acids, and phytonutrients. Do not take a green superfood in the evening since it is stimulating and may cause insomnia. However, all the ingredients are natural and contain no stimulants such as caffeine or ephedra.

Radishes

Radishes act as a natural cleanser for the digestive system by breaking down and eliminating stagnant food and toxins. Thanks to their calming effect, they can help relieve bloating and indigestion. And, with a low calorie count, they help add fiber to your diet without adversely affecting your health.[1]

Leeks

This allium vegetable similar to garlic, onions, shallots, and scallions, but with a milder flavor, can be added to everything from salads to soups. Full of fiber, they are also chock full of vitamins and such minerals as copper and iron, and are believed to contain some of the same benefits as garlic and onions.[2]

Carrots

Carrots are often referred to a superfood for the eyes because of their high content of beta-carotene. In addition, when the liver converts beta-carotene into vitamin A, it helps flush out toxins and reduce bile and fat in the liver. Plus, carrot fibers help clean out your colon and increase the movement of waste through the system.[3]

Asparagus

This vegetable is full of nutrients that help heal the gut walls. It is a good source of fiber and protein, which promote better digestion. Asparagus also contains trace minerals that boost your immunity, and a unique carb called inulin. This carb remains undigested until it reaches the large intestine, where it helps to absorb nutrients.[4]

Jerusalem artichoke

A crunchy vegetable, these artichokes are high in fiber, with soluble and insoluble kinds that help retain moisture in your gut. The roughage they provide can help reduce constipation problems and offer protection for your colon by eliminating toxic compounds. They also contain antioxidant vitamins, minerals, and electrolytes such as potassium, which can reduce blood pressure.[5]

Jicama

This member of the bean family is another excellent source of fiber, minerals, potassium, vitamins, magnesium, and antioxidants that can protect your gut against inflammation. However, while low in calories, their high carbohydrate content means you should eat them sparingly.[6]

Turmeric

Commonly found in curry powder, this healthy spice protects your liver and is a natural body cleanser. It contains a substance called curcuma, which has been used for thousands of years in the Far East to control pain and swelling in the joints. It helps the body fight inflammation and depression, which can express itself in gut-linked diseases.

Chapter 9

VITAMINS

W E HAVE EMPHASIZED the need for more fruits and vegetables as a way of improving gut health and improving your overall health by helping you ingest more natural vitamins and minerals. Yet what are Americans largely eating? Fat- and chemical-laden fast foods with no nutritional value. Not surprisingly, these nutritionally void creations make people fat faster and sick more often. Hooked on convenience, even at home too many people reach for premade dinners that originated in a factory-filled box, can, or freezer bag. These dinners have had the vitamins, minerals, and other healthy ingredients processed out of them. Meanwhile, in an effort to maximize profits, manufacturers process in preservatives, false flavorings, and fake texturizers.

If convenience foods weren't bad enough, there is the widespread American habit of eating white bread, which is bad for you in many ways. Earlier we mentioned how it lacks fiber, meaning the only thing it does for you is leave a mass of gluey glop in your stomach. Then it slowly slogs on through the digestive system and lies too long in your gut. White bread is made from bleached, or enriched (an ironic name, since that means all the nutrition has been sucked out) flour. Manufacturers then add sugar and loads of preservatives to keep that appealing but unhealthy loaf "fresh" on store shelves.

What's worse, *enriched* is a huge misnomer. Enriched flour has had most of the natural vitamins and minerals removed to give the bread a finer texture and longer shelf life. Your body absorbs it as a starch instead of a wheat or a grain, which it can use effectively for energy. Although enriched with B vitamins and iron, it lacks the vitamin E, natural fiber, and healthy trace minerals found in whole wheat flour. Goods made with this processed flour contain more empty calories than products made with whole wheat.

Eating too much sugar is another gut-busting bad habit that interferes with the absorption of vitamins and minerals crucial to healthy immune response, makes mayhem with your metabolism, and disables your neurotransmitters. The energy rush and insulin spike that you get from sugar creates an imbalanced body chemistry.

Healthy Juice

One way to obtain more vitamins through what you eat and drink is by juicing fruits and vegetables. You may have already heard of its benefits; thanks to the popular Juiceman juicer, millions are aware of the incredible amount of nourishment juicing can provide. There is a reason reducing fresh fruits and raw vegetables to juice in special combinations promotes good health. Drinking fresh juices extracted from raw fruits and vegetables furnishes all the cells in the body with the elements they need—and in a manner in which the system can easily digest and assimilate them. Fruit juices help cleanse the body, while vegetable juices build and regenerate it. Vegetable juices contain all the vitamins, minerals, salts, amino acids, and enzymes the body requires.

Another benefit of adding juices to your diet is that juices are digested and assimilated within ten to fifteen minutes of consumption. They are then utilized almost completely by the body to nourish and regenerate the cells, tissues, glands, and organs. The end result is very positive because of the minimal effort needed by the digestive system to assimilate them.

Juice isn't the only way to get more vitamins into your system. Try such foods as avocados. Despite the bad rap they sometimes get for having too much fat, avocados are amazingly healthy. They do contain up to 15 percent of the daily recommended amount of fat; however, it is good fat—the polyunsaturated and monounsaturated fat that helps to moisturize skin and keep you feeling satisfied. Avocados contain folate, which helps blood formation and is essential for cell regeneration. The oil from avocados aids in triggering the production of collagens. So incorporating more avocados into your diet will mean less wrinkles and a more even, toned skin appearance. Avocados are rich in potassium (60 percent more than bananas), vitamin A, vitamin E—an effective, fat-soluble antioxidant vital to the normalcy of body functions—and B vitamins, which help with metabolism and energy levels.

Vitamin-rich foods will not only help you achieve healthier insides, but they will also improve your outward look. To give your skin a robust vitamin C treatment from the inside out, you can eat foods extra rich in vitamin C, such as citrus fruits (oranges, grapefruits, and lemons), bell peppers (red and green), broccoli, cauliflower, and dark leafy greens (spinach, kale, and mustard greens). Vitamin B complex is also important for your skin, and is found in such foods as oatmeal and bananas.

The Need for Vitamins

Experts agree that one of the best ways to safeguard your health is to eat only the healthiest foods you can find. Plenty of fresh fruits, vegetables, and whole grains along with low-fat dairy are the general recommendation. This is because of all of the "phytochemicals," or vitamins, minerals, and fiber that are naturally occurring and health protective. However, given the stress that so many people today face from work, family, and the pressures of life in general, most experts agree that a multivitamin/mineral supplement makes perfect sense. A good vitamin supplement can close nutritional gaps left by poor dietary habits. Evidence suggests that vitamins may increase your "health span," which means active years free from chronic illness (many of which originate in the gut).

Mainstream medicine once held to the theory that you can get all of the vitamins and minerals you need from your diet. However, this idea is slowly dying out. Increasing numbers of physicians realize that while the "Greatest Generation" may have received all the nutrition they required from their foods, this is simply not the case any longer. Mineral-depleted soils and chemical agribusiness farming and marketing methods almost guarantee that you will not get anywhere near the nutritional value needed for health from foods you buy at the supermarket.

The elderly who used to be able to rely on their food can benefit from vitamins as well. One study shows that people over the age of sixty-five who take multivitamins daily suffer only half as many infection-related illnesses as people who do not take vitamins.[1] In addition, researchers believe that vitamin E, when taken at the onset of middle age, will slow damage due to aging in the human brain and immune system. Based upon a study in which middle-age mice and old-age mice were fed diets supplemented with vitamin E, results showed that normal age-related damage to vital proteins in their brains and immune system cells was delayed and even prevented.[2]

When choosing a multivitamin, it is important to remember that not all vitamins are created equal. Here are some considerations to help you make the best choices:

+ Look for the "USP" number on the label. This number gives you the percentage of the product that has been formulated to dissolve after one hour in body fluids. The percentage should be as high as possible and will vary from product to product.

+ Make sure the iron in your multivitamin is either ferrous fumarate or ferrous sulfate because they are the most absorbable forms.

+ For best absorption, take your multivitamin with meals and not on an empty stomach. Otherwise you may experience nausea.

+ Another important tip is to make sure that you take your multivitamin with a meal that contains a little fat. The fat-soluble vitamins (A, D, and E) need a little fat to get inside your system and go to work.

+ Remember that all of the B vitamins are important for normal brain and nervous system function. Taking a complex of the water-soluble B vitamins as part of your daily nutrient supplements is critical in maintaining a healthy nervous system.

Chapter 10

SUPPLEMENTS

THUS FAR, WE have reviewed lifestyle habits that can create a healthy digestive system, such as improving your diet to enhance digestion and absorption of food, proper elimination of waste, and increased intake of good bacteria. Another step involves taking natural nutritional supplements to improve digestion. In addition to helping maintain a healthy system, a supplement such as digestive enzymes can reduce the occurrence of candida in the intestines.

There are numerous supplements available, so rather than get overwhelmed by the choices, decide which are most appropriate to your condition. Draw up a plan and choose a high-quality brand of supplement as recommended by your physician, alternative health care practitioner, or trusted nutraceutical source.

Supplements are an excellent way to help your body complete its task of strengthening your system and defending it against the diseases that can invade your gut. Your body is so sophisticated that it is programmed to signal you when it needs a nutrient or a vitamin you haven't supplied. These signals come in the form of cravings. Have you ever just *had to have* a glass of orange juice? Your body was probably telling your brain that it needed more vitamin C.

Cravings can follow a meal when the body realizes that, although it's been fed, it still hasn't received enough nutrients. Too often, instead of discerning the craving properly, people fuel it with even more non-nutritious food; therefore, the cravings return, setting off a new junk food binge. The cycle becomes vicious; while you get fatter, your body suffers from a lack of real nutrition. Sound familiar? It is likely your body is slightly malnourished.

Vitamins, minerals, and supplements are vital today for the proper fueling of the body. Most old-time farmers know that for soil to supply the food it produces with enough vitamins and minerals, it must rest or lie fallow every few years. But in an era of high-tech agriculture, this no longer occurs. Therefore, much of the American food supply is depleted of the vitamins, minerals, and nutrients your body needs to maintain good health. This is where supplementation can bridge the gap.

It is important to obtain a good supply of all the various vitamins your body needs. Because most multivitamins only contain twelve vitamins in their inactive form, you may want to choose a multivitamin you can take two to three times a day. To prevent the adrenal glands from becoming exhausted, you need to supplement your diet daily with a comprehensive multivitamin and mineral formula with adequate amounts of B-complex vitamins.

Immune System Declines

Chapter 7 mentioned the autoimmune diseases that can stem from poor gut health. During the aging process, a natural decline in immune system function takes place in every person beginning as early as the thirties. This is due to a deficiency in certain nutrients throughout life. That is why every person, regardless of whether or not they are demonstrating symptoms of any of these diseases, should protect their immune system with nutritional supplements. These include the following:

- Vitamin E: The recommended dose is 800 international units (IU) daily to protect the immune system. In addition, tocotrienols are "cousins" of vitamin E and essential for vitamin E to work properly; take 105 milligrams daily.
- Vitamin C: Vitamin C is critical for lymphocyte function, which is why it is good to drink orange juice when you have a cold. Take two grams (2,000 mg) of vitamin C per day.
- Zinc: For immune system protection, use 15 mg per day. However, it is wise to use caution when taking zinc since it affects the body's absorption of copper. It is best to take zinc in the form of a multivitamin that also supplements copper. If you increase zinc intake without also increasing copper, you may become copper deficient. And because copper is necessary for white blood cell function, any deficiency will

adversely affect the immune system, which is the opposite of the effect you want to achieve. In addition, too much zinc in the system will interfere with immune system function. Take only the recommended dosages to avoid a host of unnecessary problems.

+ Beta-carotene: The body transforms beta-carotene into vitamin A, known to strengthen the immune system. Taking beta-carotene is preferable to taking higher doses of vitamin A, which can affect liver function. The body will take the beta-carotene it receives and only manufacture the vitamin A that it needs. Take 20,000 IU a day.

+ Selenium: This mineral has been known to be critical to the immune system by stimulating the "natural killer" cells that attack harmful viruses or cancers. It also balances the immune system so it can work more effectively. Take 200 micrograms (mcg) daily.

Since many people suffering from problems in their gut are also dealing with obesity or overweight conditions, another supplement to consider is 5-HTP, a naturally occurring chemical found in *Griffonia*, a plant native to India. This chemical works differently from other weight-loss products; in the body it is converted into the neurotransmitter serotonin. Prescription antidepressants that increase serotonin levels can also help certain patients lose weight. Since 5-HTP directly increases serotonin levels, it comes as no surprise that it can function as a weight-loss aid.

Though causes for weight gain and obesity are complex, they may be related—in part—to a decreased conversion of the common amino acid tryptophan to 5-HTP, which results in lowered serotonin levels. This supplement produces a feeling of satiety (satisfaction), which results from normalizing serotonin levels. Patients on 5-HTP supplements tend to get full more quickly and are not as hungry. Start with a dose of fifty to one hundred milligrams three times daily and gradually increase the dosage.

However, use caution with any supplements, especially if you are on any medications. For example, it is not safe to take 5-HTP treatments if you are taking any type of antidepressant that changes the serotonin levels in your brain, such as Prozac, Zoloft, or Celexa. If you are on a prescription blood thinner such as Coumadin, many supplements can interfere with its effectiveness. This is why, in addition to a good recommendation, you should also check with your doctor to see which supplements are safe for you to take.

Other supplements

All of the B vitamins are important for normal brain and nervous system function. Taking a complex of the water-soluble B vitamins is critical in maintaining the healthy nervous system that aids with gut health. A dose of one hundred milligrams of vitamin B_3 three times daily can be useful because of its effect on cerebral circulation. (This dosage should not be taken by those with high blood pressure or liver problems.) In addition, an extra B complex—one hundred milligrams two to three times daily—as well as extra B_6 (fifty milligrams daily) may be helpful during periods of dizziness. Up to 1,000 mcg of vitamin B_{12} daily can also be useful.

Chapter 5 reviewed the importance of fiber for a healthy gut. Among the healthy sources of fiber mentioned was oatmeal, which also has an incredible impact on the insulin levels in your bloodstream. When you eat sugary foods, the insulin converts those carbohydrates into fat storage and slows down your metabolism. But the fiber present in oatmeal blunts that insulin response. If your circumstances prevent you from fixing a bowl of oatmeal or another type of oat bran cereal for breakfast, fiber supplements such as apple pulp concentrate, citrus pectin, and glucomannan (from the konjac plant), can have the same effect.

Finally, if you are suffering from a gut disease that leaves you feeling sluggish, consider an energy booster. L-carnitine is an amino acid that helps turn food into energy by shuttling fatty acids into the mitochondria, which act as energy factories by burning fatty acids. Humans synthesize very little carnitine, which is why a supplement can help, especially with obese and older individuals, who typically have lower levels of carnitine and thus greater difficulty burning fat for energy.

Food sources of L-carnitine include milk, meat such as mutton and lamb, fish, and cheese. In supplement form, take a combination of L-carnitine and acetyl-L-carnitine, lipoic acid, PQQ (pyrroloquinoline quinone), and a glutathione-boosting supplement. The best time to take these supplements is in the morning and early afternoon on an empty stomach. If you take them any later, these supplements can impair your sleep. Green tea supplements and N-acetyl L-tyrosine also help to increase your energy.

Chapter 11

EXERCISE

As NOTED PREVIOUSLY, many people struggling with gut diseases also battle obesity or overweight conditions. While there are many factors involved, the modern American sedentary lifestyle is an obvious contributor. In the past, the hard work in an agricultural or industrial culture gave people plenty of exercise during the day; however, the modern corporate, technological culture puts far more people in front of desks and conference tables, or in meetings where they get little activity. This problem doesn't just plague adults. Too many children no longer play sports or participate in other outdoor activities. Instead they get entranced by video games, smartphones, text messaging, social networking, TV, and movies. Combined with fast food, reducing exercise to a flick of the finger on a remote control spells ever-increasing weight gain.

If such habits characterize your lifestyle, the best prescription is a simple one: get moving! There is no better way to improve gut health than physical activity. Considered the best "nutrient" of all, exercise can prolong fitness at any age, increase your stamina and circulation, lift depression, and increase joint mobility. The leading benefit for your gut is the way it enhances digestion and elimination. Activity also tones the heart and blood vessels, controls insulin production, improves the appetite, and stimulates the lymphatic system, which aids in the removal of toxic material from the body.

It even helps raise the metabolic rate (the rate of energy expended when at rest) during and after activity. This happens because it enables you to develop more muscle, which raises the metabolic rate all day—even while you sleep. And it burns off dangerous belly fat and improves your ability to cope with stress by lowering cortisol, a stress hormone. Such activity also raises serotonin levels, which helps reduce cravings for sweets and carbohydrates.

A caution: It is important to talk with your personal physician before starting any kind of exercise program. Even if you have health considerations, though, you may be surprised to learn there are many ways to become more active. Cycling, swimming, dancing, hiking, and sports—such as basketball, volleyball, soccer, and tennis—are all considered aerobic. Washing the car by hand, working in your yard, or mowing the grass qualifies too. An aerobic exercise is simply something that uses large muscle groups of the body and raises the heart rate to a range that will burn fat for fuel. This is why aerobic exercise is one of the best ways to lose body fat.

Walking to Health

Brisk walking is the simplest and most convenient way to exercise aerobically. Walk fast enough so that you can't sing, yet slow enough so that you can talk. This is a simple way to ensure you are entering your target heart rate zone. The Centers for Disease Control and Prevention (CDC) recommends brisk walking five days a week for thirty minutes. Start by walking only ten minutes a day and gradually increase your time to thirty minutes.

Diabetic patients with foot ulcers or numbness in the feet may want to avoid walking in favor of cycling, an elliptical machine, or pool activities. Aerobic exercise will make you feel better immediately by putting more oxygen into your body. Whatever activity you choose, the important thing is to get moving regularly. Don't give yourself an excuse to justify a lack of activity. As you look for ways to increase your activity level, keep these tips in mind:

+ Choose something that is fun and enjoyable. You will never stick to any program if you dread or hate it.
+ Wear comfortable, well-fitting shoes and socks.
+ If you are a type 1 diabetic, you will need to work with your doctor in order to adjust insulin doses while increasing your activity. Realize that exercising will lower your blood sugar; this can be potentially dangerous in a type 1 diabetic.

Regardless of what exercise routine you follow, remember that every activity either requires or can be performed at different levels of intensity. Given that, it makes sense that every person hoping to lose weight has an ideal intensity at which he or she should work out. This is called your target heart rate zone, which generally ranges from 65 to 85 percent of your maximum heart rate.

To calculate the low end of this zone, start by subtracting your age from 220. This is your maximum heart rate. For example, for someone forty years old the formula is: 220 - 40 = 180 beats per minute. Multiply this number by 65 percent to find the low end of the target heart rate zone: 180 x 0.65 = 117 beats per minute. To figure out the high end of the zone, multiply your maximum heart rate by 85 percent: 180 x 0.85 = 153 beats per minute. So, if you are forty, when exercising you should keep your heart rate between 117 and 153 beats per minute.

High-intensity aerobic exercise decreases insulin levels and increases levels of glucagon. By lowering insulin levels, you release more stored body fat and thus burn fat, not carbohydrates. By maintaining a moderate pace as you exercise, you will keep your body burning fat as fuel. When you exercise to the point that you are severely short of breath, you are no longer performing aerobically. Instead you have shifted to an anaerobic activity, which burns stored sugar as primary fuel instead of fat.

If you are just starting to exercise and aim to burn primarily fat, you need to work out at a moderate intensity of 65 to 85 percent of your maximum heart rate. When starting any activity program, aim for the 65 percent target, increasing gradually as you become more aerobically conditioned. Be sure that as you increase the intensity of workouts, you remain able to converse with another person.

How Much Is Enough?

The CDC and the National Institutes of Health (NIH) recommend that adults get two types of physical activity each week: aerobic and muscle-strengthening. For aerobic activity they recommend two hours and thirty minutes of moderate intensity aerobic activity (i.e., brisk walking, water aerobics, riding a bike on level ground, playing doubles tennis, or pushing a lawn mower), or one hour and fifteen minutes of vigorous exercise (jogging, swimming, riding a bike fast or on hills, playing singles tennis, or basketball). For muscle strengthening, or resistance exercise, they recommend two or more days a week, working all major muscle groups (legs, hips, back, abdomen, chest, shoulders, and arms).[1]

If you can only do moderate intensity activities, try brisk walking for thirty minutes a day, five days a week. If you can handle more vigorous activity, jog for twenty-five minutes a day, three days a week. Or you can break it down even further: five days a week, try going for a ten-minute walk three times a day.

If you are not sure you are getting enough activity, try monitoring the steps you walk with a pedometer. Typically a person walks three thousand to five thousand steps a day. To stay fit, set a goal of ten thousand steps, or approximately five miles. Before engaging in any activity, make sure that you have either eaten a meal two or three hours prior or have had a healthy snack about thirty to sixty minutes beforehand. It is never good to work out when hungry; you may end up burning muscle protein as energy, which is very expensive fuel.

If you have a condition such as arthritis, you may be hesitant to start an exercise program. When you are in pain, you don't want to "rock the boat" and make things worse. This calls for reasonable steps, such as practicing deep breathing exercises daily; outdoors in the morning is especially good. Stretching exercises will help to limber up your body in the morning; stretching before going to bed at night will help to relax you and promote more restful sleep. Even with arthritis, you can start a walking program, starting slowly. As you continue, you will likely be able to walk faster and for longer periods of time.

Daily Activity Journal

If your battle with gut diseases includes a struggle with too much weight, consider taking steps to monitor your activity. Researchers say that self-monitoring devices, such as a pedometer, heart rate monitor, or even a simple exercise journal, can account for a 25 percent increase in successfully controlling your weight.[2] A good activity journal should monitor your waist measurement, body fat percentage, what you eat, and how often you exercise.

For additional motivation, find a photograph of yourself at or near a healthy or desired weight and put it in your food journal. Or, if you don't have one handy, take a "before" picture of yourself now and an "after" when you reach a certain goal. Whichever photo you use, as you carry your journal throughout the day, visualize yourself becoming an ideal weight again.

In case you need a reminder, here are some of the many benefits that regular activity promotes:

- It improves digestion, a key for a healthy gut.
- It alleviates pain and gives you more restful sleep.
- It decreases the risk of heart disease, stroke, and the development of hypertension, and helps prevent type 2 diabetes.
- It helps prevent osteoporosis and aids in maintaining healthy bones.
- It slows down the aging process, helps prevent arthritis, and aids in maintaining healthy joints.
- It improves your mood and reduces the symptoms of anxiety and depression.

Chapter 12

WONDERFUL WATER

FOR PEOPLE DEALING with poor gut health, there is no better tonic than to increase your intake of water. This precious liquid cleanses the body inside and out by transporting nutrients, proteins, vitamins, minerals, and sugars for assimilation. It helps the body to get rid of waste products, improve elimination, regulate body temperature, and act as a shock absorber for joints, bones, and muscles. In addition, water helps speed up the detoxification process, which we will discuss in greater detail in chapter 14. Keeping your body properly hydrated each day ensures optimal functioning of every organ system. When you drink enough water, your body works at peak performance.

Water is particularly vital for anyone dealing with internal toxicity. While this condition has several causes, among them are constipation and a lack of water to help flush toxins out of your system. Water also speeds up the digestive and eliminative processes. Failing to eliminate toxins through regular bowel movements means they just recirculate into the bloodstream and make your condition worse. Adding more water (and fiber) to your diet will improve the condition of your gut.

There are obvious symptoms of an unhealthy digestive tract: poor digestion, lower backache, fatigue, body odor, gas, and stomach bloating, to name a few. Add the psychological load of stress and it spells hindered food digestion, absorption, and elimination. The end result is an unhealthy colon and other health problems. In fact, many Americans suffer from aches and pains, constipation, skin eruptions, and fatigue. Often a lack of water is the root cause. Our society consumes coffee by the gallon and soft drinks and iced tea by the liter. Plain old water is boring or distasteful for some people.

Many people mistakenly believe that because they drink large quantities of iced tea, coffee, concentrated juices, and soft drinks, they are getting plenty of liquid nourishment. Wrong! Your body simply cannot function properly without pure water. Drinking plenty of pure (not tap) water every day will keep you hydrated and your body's systems working more efficiently.

DEHYDRATION HAZARDS

Water makes up 65 to 75 percent of the human body and is second only to oxygen as an essential need for survival. In fact, your brain is more than 80 percent water, and your blood is more than 90 percent water. Through breathing, urination, and sweating, you lose approximately sixty-four ounces of water a day. This means you need to drink eight eight-ounce glasses of water just to break even and replenish yourself. Few people drink enough water to break even, meaning millions of people are chronically dehydrated. People who suffer from problems with water retention, edema (swelling), and bloating are simply not drinking enough water. Once they do, these symptoms improve.

Do you often feel fatigued, irritable, depressed, confused, or beset by intense food cravings? You could simply be dehydrated. You can do a couple of easy self-tests to check. First, lightly pinch the skin on the back of your hand together and pull upward. If your skin doesn't immediately recede back into place when you let go, but stays raised for a few seconds, you need more water. Second, check the color of your urine. It should be light, not dark or yellow. If your urine is colored, you need to drink more water.

Dehydration creates a multitude of physical problems. It gives illness and disease a chance to take hold in your body. Many illnesses are exacerbated by, or even result from, chronic dehydration. Often, when your doctor diagnoses an illness, you're not so much *sick* as you are *thirsty*. The medical community often ends up treating the effects of pitifully low water intake with medication. However, many medications can poison your body and generate undesirable side effects, so you want to avoid them as much as possible. In large part, you can accomplish that by drinking the water your body so desperately needs. A well-hydrated body is a healthy body.

If you significantly increase your water intake, your sensitivity to your body's need for water will also multiply. The more water you give your body, the more you will know when you need it. That is a good way to start a healthy cycle. Water is the ultimate detoxifier. If you aren't getting enough, an increase of only five glasses a day can improve your gut health, as well as fight cancer. In fact, adequate water intake can cut the risk of colon cancer by 45 percent, bladder cancer by 50 percent, and breast cancer by 79 percent. Cancer can only develop in an acidic environment, and dehydration causes your body to be acidic.

Many people live on the cusp of acidity—a real risk to health—but the more water you drink, the more balanced your pH levels. Water also acts as a powerful cleanser to remove plaque from artery walls. It is instrumental in stabilizing blood pressure. In addition, water lubricates the joints to prevent arthritis and diminishes headaches. Dehydration can cause all kinds of painful symptoms; water can decrease them all, or even make them disappear.

WATER SOURCES

If you have not been drinking water and eight glasses a day seems like a lot, start slowly and gradually increase your intake. Add a slice of fresh lemon, and you will get even more of a cleansing benefit. Once people catch the importance of the idea, the next concern is what kind of water they should be drinking. This is a valid concern. Most municipal tap water supplies are chlorinated, fluoridated, or otherwise chemically treated to the point of being an irritant to the system instead of a blessing. Also, many toxic chemicals have found their way into ground water, adding more pollutants to the water supply. This growing concern about water purity has led to the huge bottled water industry. Many stores today have whole aisles dedicated to different kinds of bottled water, which can create confusion for the consumer.

It may help to clarify the main types of water that are offered.

First, there is mineral water, which most often comes from a natural spring with naturally occurring minerals. It has a taste that varies from one spring to the next. Naturally occurring minerals found in mineral water help to aid digestion and bowel function. Europeans have long recognized the benefits of bottled mineral water. California and Florida regulate the purity of mineral water produced in their states.

Second, there is distilled water. You may have known someone who believes that drinking distilled water is the only way to go. While distilled water is probably the purest water available, it is also demineralized. On a long-term basis, this is not ideal, since the body needs the minerals that naturally occur in water. This lack of minerals detracts from its qualities as a good cleanser and detoxifier. If you are on a detoxifying program or on chemotherapy, distilled water is excellent to remove debris and toxins. Once finished, return to drinking a good mineral or spring water to ensure proper mineral activity.

Sparkling water is another choice that comes from natural carbonation in underground springs. Most varieties are artificially boosted in carbonation by CO_2 to maintain a longer fizz. Many people enjoy sparkling water after dinner as an aid to digestion.

If you choose not to purchase bottled water, you can purify your water by using a water filter in your home. You can purchase water filters that attach to your kitchen sink faucet and remove impurities as water flows out of the tap. You may also have noticed that some water pitchers contain filters that purify the water as you fill the pitcher. Both methods are necessary to help improve the quality of the water you consume.

Whatever type of water you choose, to maintain good gut health the most important thing to remember is to pay conscious attention to getting your quota of water every day. Thirst is not a reliable signal that your body needs water. You can easily lose a quart or more of water during activity before you even feel thirsty. Also remember that caffeine and alcohol are diuretics, which increase your body's need for water. If you consume caffeine or alcohol, make sure you drink enough water to compensate.

Chapter 13

ACID REFLUX

A CID REFLUX DISEASE (reflux esophagitis) is a digestive disorder of epidemic proportions, with one of every ten Americans suffering from its symptoms. It is caused by the stomach acid refluxing up into the esophagus, which occurs when the valve (the esophageal sphincter) does not close properly. Thus, stomach juices back up into the esophagus. Overeating or eating foods that relax the lower muscles of the esophagus can cause reflux. Other causes include a diet high in junk, fast, and processed foods, and overuse of medications.

While periodic episodes of heartburn caused by acid reflux are common, when they occur frequently they can become much more than a nuisance. Frequent occurrences of episodes of acid reflux (technically known as *gastroesophageal reflux disease*, or GERD) can increase the potential risk of esophageal cancer by causing changes in the cells lining the esophagus. So instead of just shrugging it off or grumbling about this irritation ruining your sleep last night, take action.

You may wonder: When does heartburn constitute a serious enough problem that you should seek help? If you are consistently having more than three episodes of heartburn weekly, you should consult your doctor. Don't allow these symptoms to continue long term. People who ignore the problem in hopes it will just go away can develop scar tissue in the esophagus. This scar tissue narrows the esophagus, which can cause major difficulties and even require surgical correction.

Still, don't automatically reach for a traditional pill solution. Prilosec, the prescription (and now available in over-the-counter form) used to treat it, is one of the top-selling drugs in the world. You may already be spending a small fortune on such remedies to deal with your digestive problems. The trouble with that is that symptoms are only a signal, a way your body communicates that something is not right. Antacids may make you feel better temporarily, but this doesn't address the root cause.

Besides masking symptoms and ignoring what your body is trying to tell you, this can cause health problems to escalate.

Home Remedy for Acid Reflux

There are some commonsense remedies to help you if you are suffering from acid reflux, starting with avoiding antacids. An overly acidic stomach does not cause heartburn. Maalox, Rolaids, Mylanta, and other antacids contain aluminum, while Tums and others contain calcium. Both aluminum and calcium can increase acidity, causing further discomfort and the need for more antacids. In addition, aluminum is linked to Alzheimer's disease.

Other things to avoid include the following:

- Prescription-strength and over-the-counter medications, such as Pepcid AC, Prilosec, Tagamet, Zantac, and the like. They block normal body processes, impair proper digestion of food, and impede mineral absorption. Long-term use of these medications can damage the stomach lining and increase the risk of benign and cancerous tumors.
- Stress and anger
- Estrogen (e.g., birth control pills and menopause treatments), which can cause the lower muscles of the esophagus to weaken
- Smoking, which aggravates heartburn

Fooling your body never fixes anything. Your digestive system takes charge of a miraculously interactive process that releases and absorbs nutrients from the foods you eat, which are needed for healthy living. In the mouth, enzymes in saliva begin breaking down food. In the stomach, acid and enzymes break down food and release vitamins, minerals, protein, and fats.

Pancreatic juices and bile from the gallbladder get in on the act too.

A phenomenal relationship between the brain and gut takes place on a molecular level as neuropeptides and serotonins guide absorption of the released nutrients traveling through the intestines. Without well-absorbed nutrients, none of the body's systems can enjoy optimum health. When the digestive system is out of balance, it belches, burns, cramps, or explodes. It is important to listen to what your body is trying to tell you, not shut it up with prescription drugs or over-the-counter remedies.

Adjust Your Eating

Most remedies for acid reflux and heartburn reduce stomach acid. Now, acid isn't always a bad thing. A car battery can't function without acid; your digestive system can't either. The stomach acid breaks down foods and releases essential nutrients into the body. Furthermore, reducing stomach acid leaves the stomach at the mercy of germs and bacteria that cause food poisoning and other maladies.

Laboratory studies in rats have demonstrated that antioxidants from fresh fruits and vegetables can do more to heal acid reflux than prescription medications! So dealing with this disease starts with eating habits. Change your diet to include 75 percent raw foods (fruits, vegetables, and whole grains). Eat smaller amounts of food too, and more often, to avoid pressure in the abdomen. Avoid such offenders as fried foods, soft drinks, chocolate, coffee, and alcohol.

Foods to Avoid if You Are Fighting Reflux

This chapter talks about avoiding coffee, chocolate, and peppermint. But there are other foods or habits that can increase acid reflux symptoms. Here are some other things you should avoid:

- Alcohol
- High-fat foods
- Drinking excessive fluids with a meal (it is important not to drink over four ounces of fluid with a meal,

> since excess fluid will increase tendencies to have
> reflux if the valve is not functioning properly)
>
> - In addition, try drinking between a half-quart and a
>   quart of aloe vera juice throughout the day. Beware
>   of drinking too much, though, since it can lead to
>   diarrhea.

In addition to adjusting the kinds of food you eat, eat large meals early and light meals later in the day. Years ago people tended to eat larger meals in the early part of the day and lighter meals in the evening. In the modern, hyper-speed age, this typical pattern has been reversed. Many people skip breakfast, eat a small lunch, and consume their largest meal in the evening. This is the opposite of the way God designed your body to function. Not too surprisingly, while America's eating patterns have changed, the rate of obesity increased. The combination of these factors has produced increasing problems with esophageal disease.

There is a muscular valve, known as a *sphincter*, between the esophagus and the stomach. The lining of the stomach is designed to handle a high acid level, but if this acid "refluxes"—or backs up—into the esophagus, it can cause problems. The cells lining the esophagus are not designed to handle high acid levels. Acid can cause severe damage and even erosions and inflammation in the esophagus, which can produce heartburn symptoms.

When you eat late in the evening, it leaves large amounts of food in the stomach when you go to bed, producing pressure on the sphincter muscle. If you are carrying extra pounds, it produces additional pressure on the stomach, which in turn causes more acid to enter the esophagus. The simple habit of eating a light meal early in the evening can dramatically reduce these symptoms.

FIVE NATURAL STEPS

Granted, serious cases of acid reflux may require prescription medications to protect you from the dire consequences of this disease. Before going that route, though, there are five helpful suggestions that have been proven to quench heartburn without prescription medicine. The first we've already reviewed: eating larger meals earlier in the day. The other four simple, at-home techniques you can try before seeking medical help are as follows:

1. Raise the head of your bed.

   A small block of wood such as a two-by-four (or even a four-by-four) block placed under the head of the bed can elevate the entire bed. This prevents the return of acid into the esophagus and helps contain the acid in the stomach, where it belongs. Adding an extra pillow or two under your head can actually make the problem worse because of the angle created between the esophagus and the stomach.

2. Avoid the three "bad guys"—peppermint candy, coffee, and chocolate.

   These three certain substances can weaken the tone or strength of the sphincter muscle, allowing acid to reflux. Ironically, after a meal at a restaurant, many people reach for a cup of coffee, a peppermint candy, or a chocolate mint. You would be wise to resist.

3. Drink more water.

   The previous chapter reviewed the need for water to flush the system and keep you hydrated, but increasing your daily consumption of water is also a simple, effective remedy for heartburn. Why? Water tends to wash the acid off the wall of the esophagus.

4. Use antacids with caution.

   If you need to use an occasional antacid, remember liquid antacids are better than tablets because they tend to adhere to the esophagus and form a protective coating. There are over-the-counter medications known as H2 blockers, which include Tagamet and similar medications; these can be used on occasion, but as your grow older, the stomach tends to produce less acid. The chronic use of these medications to neutralize acid can sometimes interfere with digestion.

Whichever method or methods you use, don't allow symptoms to continue for long before seeing a physician.

Peppermint Oil

If you are suffering from irritable bowel syndrome as well as acid reflux, an effective natural treatment for IBS is enteric-coated peppermint oil. Research has indicated that the oil found in the peppermint plant can relax smooth muscles in the colon. Prescription muscle relaxants (known as *antispasmodics*) can cause numerous side effects, but the peppermint oil found in the plant kingdom has no side effects.[1] There is one small problem with peppermint oil, which we mentioned earlier: peppermint can be a major irritant of acid reflux. This makes it imperative that you take the coated capsule form of the peppermint oil so that the oil will be absorbed in the intestine rather than in the stomach.

Still, researchers have seen excellent results with the use of peppermint oil. It tends to stop the excessive spasms in the smooth muscles and helps maintain the muscle tone in the colon. Peppermint oil capsules have been used for several years in Europe for the treatment of IBS and have been found to be very safe and effective. Researchers in Britain recorded a nearly 50 percent reduction in colon spasms after peppermint oil was introduced into the colon. The capsules are available in a standardized, coated form that contains 0.2 milliliters of peppermint oil.

Chapter 14

HEALTHY GUT DETOXES

SINCE THE LIVER processes everything you eat, drink, or absorb through your skin, it accumulates toxins in the same way a car accumulates grime, dust, and wear and tear. Just as a car needs an engine tune-up, filters, and hoses, your body's filter—the liver—needs periodic flushing and cleaning. (Ironically, many people take better care of their cars than their physical bodies.) Detoxification is a way to cleanse your gut and rid it of toxins and debris you have accumulated over the years. This provides a clean foundation on which you can build for the future.

How do you know if you need to detoxify? Here are some indicators:

+ You suffer from poor elimination.
+ The majority of your diet is junk food and sugar.
+ You are involved in overeating, stress eating, or late-night eating (or a combination).
+ You suffer from fatigue and stress-related aches, pains, and rashes.
+ You take antibiotics often and don't get much exercise.

If you relate to several of these symptoms, detoxification will be a blessing and give you the best start to a stronger immune response. You may want to also consider colonic treatments; while beneficial, though, they are not essential. If you choose to start a cleansing program with colonics, supplement your intestinal tract with a bowel flora formula such as acidophilus or bifidus. Colonics can strip healthy bowel flora along with the toxins and encrusted matter in the intestines.

If colonic treatments do not appeal, try using Nature's Secret Ultimate Cleanse by Lindsey Duncan. It can help those who struggle with poor bowel function and digestive difficulties. This two-part program cleanses channels of elimination, including your liver, kidneys, and colon. It will take about thirty days to consume the two bottles provided in the program. During that time you must drink plenty of non-chlorinated water and eat a diet that is as close to the "garden" as possible. This means things such as organic fruits, vegetables, and meats. And no preservatives or refined sugars (cakes, pies, candy), caffeine, colas, dairy, alcohol, or wheat. This cleansing product offers immediate results by gently supporting the body's natural eliminative processes of two or three daily bowel movements.

Detoxing isn't just taking a few supplements or products. It is necessary to adjust your eating habits for more than thirty days. Work to establish a long-term habit of avoiding fried, sugary, and fatty foods, while eating fresh vegetables and fruits, and drinking fresh fruit juices to detoxify your body and neutralize its acidity.

Colon Health

If you do a colon cleanse, while in your detox phase, take an acidophilus supplement daily, such as Kyo-Dophilus by Wakunaga. Also, buy a loofah, a natural bristle skin brush, and brush your skin (always moving away from the heart) before showering each day. This will assist the elimination process for toxins being released through the skin. You should also drink at least six to eight glasses of pure water daily and include mild exercise, such as walking, stretching, or bike riding.

You can also enjoy a salt and soda bath. This bath counteracts the effects of radiation, whether from X-rays, cancer treatment radiation, fallout from the atmosphere, or television radiation. Simply add one cup of baking soda and one to two cups of ordinary coarse salt, Epsom salts, or sea salt to a tub of warm water. Soak for up to twenty minutes.

Once you have cleansed your colon, consider these supplements:

- Magnesium: 400 mg daily
- Continue with Kyo-Dophilus or Bio-K to replenish the intestinal tract with healthy bowel flora

- Digestive enzyme with every meal
- Milk thistle extract for liver function
- Colon Clenz by Natural Balance, Inc., for occasional bowel sluggishness
- Nature's Secret Ultimate Oil to prevent constipation

Fresh juice is especially helpful. In addition to water and easily absorbed protein and carbohydrates, fresh juice provides essential fatty acids, vitamins, minerals, enzymes, and phytonutrients. Every time you pour a glass, picture a big vitamin-mineral cocktail with a wealth of nutrients. The veggies are broken down into an easily absorbable form, promoting vitality. Since it doesn't have to go through a process of breaking everything down, juice goes to work immediately to give you energy and renew you, right down to the cellular level. Since it spares your organs the work it takes to digest food, this equates to more energy. Juice also detoxifies your body because it is rich in antioxidants, which lightens your load. The body doesn't have to work so hard to deal with all the toxic stuff.

Cleansing Symptoms

If you have never implemented a detoxification program, realize that as your body begins to "clean house" you could develop such symptoms as headaches, flu, aches and pains, nausea, or skin eruptions. Though unpleasant, these are all positive signs that the cleansing process is working. After a few weeks on a detoxification program, your mind will be clearer, your energy will soar, and both your digestion and sleep will improve. In essence, you will feel like a new person (because you are).

During this initial phase, the energy in the periphery or external parts of your body, such as the muscles and skin, moves to the vital internal organs and starts the regeneration and reconstruction process. This shunting of much of the power to the internal region produces a feeling of less energy, which the mind interprets as weakness. In reality, the body's energy is increased, but most of it is being used for rebuilding the important internal organs. That leaves less energy for the muscles.

Be assured that what you are feeling is not weakness, but a refocusing of energy to the more important internal parts. During this phase do not give in to the temptation to increase feelings of energy by taking a stimulant, since this will defeat the regeneration process. At first, as you omit such toxic substances as coffee, tea, chocolate, tobacco, excess salt, and alcohol, a headache of letdown often occurs. This usually lasts about forty-eight hours, but is followed by a feeling of well-being and strength. It is important to be patient. After a while, you will gain more strength than you had prior to this makeover program. During this phase, however, you should rest and relax, limit social obligations, and take it easy at work until the weakness passes.

As you continue this cleansing process and introduce higher-quality foods while eliminating lower-quality foods, remarkable things happen to the body as well as the mind. With higher quality food, your body begins to discard the lower grade materials to make room for the new, superior materials. Your body will choose the best materials you give it to make new and healthier tissue. It always tries to produce health and always succeeds—unless your interference overwhelms it. This self-curing nature of the body is evident in many conditions, such as the common cold, fevers, cuts, swellings, and bruises.

As your body builds up energy, you may experience more unpleasant symptoms. This newly found energy is being used to discard toxic waste, cellular debris, and poisons that cause negative symptoms for a while. It helps to understand that your body is becoming younger and healthier every day because you are throwing off more and more waste that eventually would have brought pain, disease, and much suffering.

Overcoming Yeast Infections

A detox is particularly beneficial if your body has a buildup of yeast and bacteria. One of the most important means of detoxifying the body is to have regular bowel movements on a daily basis, which means eating plenty of fiber and drinking plenty of water. As mentioned in chapter 5, you need at least twenty-five to thirty-five grams of fiber every day. With yeast overgrowths, fiber helps to eliminate yeast so that it is not reabsorbed back into the body.

During the first week of a candida program, candida die-off reactions usually occur. When a yeast cell dies, it becomes food for another yeast cell, which tends to encourage the yeast colonies that are still present. The internal fluids of the dead yeast cells are feeding these colonies; therefore, it is critically important to eliminate these dead yeast cells through adequate fiber intake.

Chlorophyll supplements, otherwise known as green food supplements, detoxify the colon and pack a powerful punch while boosting the immune system. Chlorophyll keeps yeast and bacteria from spreading, and it encourages the growth of friendly bacteria. High-chlorophyll foods include wheat grass, barley grass, alfalfa, chlorella, spirulina, and blue-green algae. These high-chlorophyll foods are nutrient dense and are excellent sources of essential amino acids, vitamins, minerals, essential fatty acids, and phytonutrients. High-chlorophyll foods boost the immune system and help to improve both digestion and elimination.

Not only does candida overgrowth affect the immune system and gastrointestinal tract, but it also has a profound impact on the liver as well. While liver detoxification occurs continually in the body, many times the body's detoxification pathways are overwhelmed by yeast, toxins produced by yeast, leaky gut syndrome, or food allergies. Therefore, herbs and supplements are critically important for supporting and improving liver detoxification. Some that will help include the following:

+ N-acetyl cysteine, otherwise known as NAC, and taurine (500 mg of each daily). These supplements will help replenish glutathione stores, which protect the liver from damage from drugs and other toxins.

+ Milk thistle, which contains a bioflavonoid called silymarin that also protects the liver against toxins.

+ Lipoic acid, which will also increase levels of glutathione.

Chapter 15

FOOD SENSITIVITIES

TODAY'S GENERATION IS different from any other in history. Instead of eating food as it naturally comes from the earth, Americans eat food that is often highly processed or tainted by multiple herbicides and pesticides. Ironically, amid our supposed progress, recent discoveries show the wisdom of the health and nutritional laws God gave to the Israelites. Though thousands of years old, they are some of the most advanced guidelines for avoiding plagues and disease ever developed. The foods God instructed the Israelites to eat in the Old Testament contain curative properties, or substances that can prevent or even reverse disease. And the "unclean" animals He forbade them to eat still carry the most dangerous bacteria and risk of disease.

So what does all this have to do with food allergies and sensitivities? Food allergies have increased several hundredfold in the past decade or so; fatal allergic reactions seem to be far more common than ever. Indeed, food allergies are fast becoming as common as a cold or flu, and have been linked to chronic fatigue. The primary cause is all the chemically altered, injected, sprayed, and dyed foods that people ingest. Stress, lack of sleep, and enzyme deficiency from foods zapped by microwave preparation make the problem worse. Other causes include an allergy to gluten-containing foods, inherited food sensitivities, MSG, sulfites, and nitrates in foods. Then there are food additives, which are designed to enhance color and flavor, but cause a myriad of problems for sensitive individuals.

Easily a quarter (probably more) of the American population exhibit allergies, including the vast majority of all children with autism, ADHD, and asthma. People are allergic to numerous substances. Among them are inhalants, such as plant pollen, animal dander, mold spores, and vehicle exhaust; and the fumes of chemical products, such as paint and cleaning solutions. People react to insect stings, antibiotics, and many drugs. Some people have allergic reactions to touching certain plants, wearing jewelry made of certain substances, and using makeup or other beauty products.

Food allergies are emerging as more significant than previously thought, especially allergies to peanuts, shellfish, eggs, and milk. And when people aren't allergic to something, they often have sensitivities to or intolerances for it.

Food Definitions

While people often lump food allergies, sensitivities, and intolerances (like the common problem of intolerance to the lactose in milk), they are not identical. To summarize:

+ A food allergy is an autoimmune system body response to a certain food or an enzyme deficiency to digest a certain food. This exaggerated response to specific substances normally poses no serious threats to the human body.
+ A sensitivity is any adverse reaction in the body that comes from exposure to a sensitizing agent in the environment. A sensitivity can involve antibodies and other immune processes. Food and chemical reactions are sensitivities.
+ An intolerance is a reaction to food that does not involve the immune system. An intolerance presupposes the absence of a particular chemical or physiologic process needed to digest a food substance. For example, the lack of a digestive enzyme may result in a food intolerance.

If you are dealing with symptoms from such problems—such as irritability, headaches, candida, gas, constipation, sinus problems, or irritable bowel syndrome—try the following for a couple of weeks to help identify the problem. Eat brown rice; baked or broiled turkey, chicken or fish; herbal teas; steamed, broiled, raw, or baked vegetables; vegetable and unsweetened, diluted fruit juices. Also add yogurt to your diet.

Keep a food diary. After two weeks, add foods back and rotate your meals. Repeat foods only once every four days. For example, if you have a tomato stuffed with tuna on Monday, you should not have it again until Friday. This way you will be able to identify a food that you are sensitive to by evaluating symptoms. Continue to keep your food diary. As you rotate and eliminate, you will feel more energy, stabilize your weight, and experience a renewed feeling of well-being.

Also, avoid these common allergy foods: peanuts, corn, mushrooms, eggs, wheat, soy, dairy, coffee, sugar, and strawberries.

Disease Links

If gut-related problems include the illness that literally "takes your breath away," you aren't alone. Asthma is a severe respiratory allergy reaction and the most serious chronic illness among children under the age of ten. It is estimated that 3 to 5 percent of the US population is affected by this disorder. There has been a 50 percent increase in diagnosed cases in the last several years, with a suspected link to the increase of environmental pollutants.[1]

Studies show that there are common triggers that precipitate an attack of asthma in children. While the most common trigger is stress, certain food allergies can also trigger it. So can such factors as food dyes, smoke, molds, pet dander, chemical toxins, and respiratory infections. In adults, asthma triggers or precipitators include adrenal gland exhaustion, constipation (another reason to eat plenty of fiber and drink lots of pure water), low thyroid function, and hypoglycemia.

Asthma sufferers should consider going on a largely vegetarian diet. Green leafy vegetables are especially good because of their high magnesium content, which helps to relax bronchial muscles. Drink plenty of water with lemon to thin mucous secretions. In order to identify your particular food sensitivities, consider allergy testing. This will help you avoid your personal triggers, thereby reducing the frequency of attacks. Reduce sodium and starchy foods in your diet. Asthmatics have more frequent attacks when they consume high amounts of sodium (salty) foods. To cut down on mucus production, avoid dairy products. Avoid soft drinks, caffeine, fried foods, sulfites, MSG, and sugary foods.

Other problems caused by food allergies include colitis and Crohn's diseases. (Refer to chapter 6 for more information on both.) Of particular concern for children are earaches. This painful condition can be caused by several factors, such as the residual effect of a bronchial infection, flu, or cold that has settled in the ear. However, other causes include food allergies (especially to dairy) and eating too many mucus-producing foods. In adults, the most common cause of earache is swimmer's ear, which involves the outer ear canal. Children frequently suffer from middle ear infections and are placed on powerful antibiotics. This in turn may cause thrush or candidiasis. Breast-feeding your children helps to safeguard them against ear infections by boosting immunity and preventing allergies.

If you or your child is suffering from an earache, eliminate all dairy, fruit juice, fried foods, milk, and sugars from the diet. Read all food labels and avoid additives such as MSG. Drink eight to ten glasses of water daily. Also have a green drink each day. Supplements that are helpful include grapefruit seed extract capsules, vitamin C, beta-glucan, and echinacea extract. For swimmer's ear, mix an ounce of distilled white vinegar and 70 percent isopropyl alcohol in a dropper bottle. Place three drops into the ear canal and then let it drain (repeat two times daily).

The Four A's

If your child suffers from one of the "four A's"—autism, attention deficit disorder (whether ADD or ADHD), asthma, or allergies—you should know that food allergies, sensitivities, and intolerances are common in these patients. Successful implementation of treatment programs is often hampered by the "picky eater" nature of these children.

You will find a range of sometimes conflicting information about diets for 4-A children. Some initial food-related testing must be done on every child while your doctor develops a treatment plan. Further testing along the way will be necessary to monitor outcomes. You should implement a diet plan based on your understanding of your child's individual metabolic problems. The actual diets themselves end up being experimental in nature, because only by using them can you determine which combination will most benefit your child at any given time.

Despite the body's incredible ability to heal itself, today's health and food environments raise formidable challenges for children. Since every child is a unique individual, both the causes of his or her particular problems and the solutions are uniquely individual. Nutrition, along with detoxification, supplements, and medications, need to be orchestrated in a tailored program. Since each healing factor has an effect on the others, they work synergistically, each amplifying the effects of the others. When combined, they are designed to heal the digestive system, which will help to eliminate major sources of toxicity in the body.

Chapter 16

END EMOTIONAL EATING

THERE IS A link between what you eat and how you feel, a causation you shouldn't overlook as you seek to improve your gut health. This starts with recognizing the possibility that you are emotionally dependent on food for comfort during times of stress, crisis, anxiety, loneliness, or a host of other emotions. You should also realize that the result of the traditional Western lifestyle is often a constant, treadmill-like cycle that keeps you feeling sluggish and frustrated. No matter what you have tried in the past, this affects your motivation to revitalize your gut and jump-start a healthier lifestyle. When you fail to achieve a breakthrough in this vital area, it negatively affects the belief that you can pursue other lifelong dreams.

When weighed down, your mind can shift into "autopilot" mode. Instead of striving to improve, you settle for the ordinary. Getting stuck in this kind of rut can affect your mind as well as your body. For example, almost every overweight person who gets tested has a sluggish, clogged liver. The causes are many, but some primary culprits are poor gut health, such as a clogged colon or candida yeast overgrowth. Some other causes are the use of prescription and OTC drugs, use of artificial sweeteners, and eating non-organic, toxic foods. A clogged liver causes your body to rapidly store high levels of body fat. Thus, metabolism slows, which contributes significantly to weight gain. And the heavier you are, the worse you feel.

One reason for listing non-organic, toxic foods is their adverse effects on your digestive system. Non-organic foods or those that have been pasteurized or cooked—anything heated more than 180 degrees for at least thirty minutes—have no enzymes. Even with vegetables, most people cook them and thus never get needed enzymes and nutrients. Without enough enzymes you will experience trouble digesting food, low metabolism, frequent gas, constipation, and bloating.

Danger of Dead Food

Unnatural and processed substances are dead foods lacking natural energy. They drain you and make you feel less energized. Such sluggish feelings will lead to feeling grouchy and expressing negative thoughts and negative speech. Eventually, what you eat will affect your thoughts. In a vicious cycle, your thoughts will then affect what you eat.

For instance, a lack of an amino acid called tryptophan can lead to depression. Tryptophan is found in raw, high-protein foods such as goji berries, spirulina, chlorella, blue-green algae, maca root, cacao, and other raw foods. Through cooking, tryptophan is destroyed, as it is sensitive to heat. Meats contain this amino acid, but if you eat only cooked meat and potatoes (a bad combination for your digestive system), the amino acid is destroyed. Incorporate raw foods into your diet and see the difference it makes in your mental outlook.

While you are trying to achieve a level of supernatural health, avoid fast-food restaurants, whether regional or national chains. Fast food is typically loaded with trans fats, highly processed sugars and fructose corn syrup, the flavor additive MSG, artificial corn sweeteners, and nitrates. Meats and dairy from fast-food and many national chain restaurants are full of growth hormones, antibiotics, and other drugs. These highly processed foods are often microwaved and lack fiber. Companies create foods to increase hunger and cause addictions, which can lead to depression and weight gain.

Emotional Balance

If you are suffering from anxiety or emotional issues that are manifesting themselves in your gut, try Anxiety Control 24. This is an amino acid support formula that contains amino acids, herbs, vitamins, and minerals, along with essential cofactors to help relax the anxious mind or stressed body. It contains the herbs passionflower and Primula officinalis, which support an overstressed body and calm the central nervous system naturally. It is a formula that can be used day or night to

fill the deficiencies caused by a stressful life. It is also wonderful for anxious or active teens.

Change your diet so you eat more raw foods and fresh, raw salads,
and drink fresh juices made of raw veggies. This will help correct an
enzyme deficiency. It will also promote better digestion and metabolism. As you start your diet, add some enzyme tablets to your meals.
If you are overweight, past consumption of highly refined or pasteurized foods, prescription and OTC drugs, and a clogged liver and colon
will hinder your ability to create enough enzymes to digest food properly. These supplements will help restore normalcy.

Skip the Sugar

Although we have previously mentioned the dangers of sugar, it is worth
noting that too often during times of stress, depression, and anxiety,
many people reach for their favorite comfort food. Such items are usually full of sugar. In the long-term, this response is detrimental to gut
health and especially to brain and body functions. In addition, rather
than quieting anxious feelings, excessive sugar consumption increases
them. If that weren't bad enough, it has been shown to suppress the
body's immune response, which can lead to disease.

For example, if you are consuming too much sugar on a daily basis,
you may be setting yourself up for low blood sugar (hypoglycemia). Even
small blood sugar fluctuations disturb your sense of well-being. Larger
fluctuations caused by consuming too much sugar cause feelings of
depression, anxiety, mood swings, fatigue, and even aggressive behavior.

Symptoms of anxiety and depression closely parallel many of the
symptoms of hypoglycemia, such as rapid pulse, crying spells, heart pal-
pitations, cold sweats, or fatigue. If these symptoms are familiar, it is
possible you are suffering from low blood sugar. To help restore normal
blood sugar levels, focus on eating more fiber and protein foods at each
meal and cutting back on simple sugars. Eat a protein snack between
meals to help keep your blood sugar levels stable all day.

It is wise to make the effort to balance your blood sugar, because low blood sugar can predispose you to developing diabetes later in life. Diabetes occurs when the body does not properly utilize the sugar and carbohydrates consumed. Because of years of abuse, the pancreas is no longer able to produce adequate insulin, which creates the condition of high blood sugar. This can be dangerous. According to the National Institute of Diabetes and Digestive and Kidney Diseases more than seventeen million people suffer from diabetes in this country.[1] Diabetes can lead to heart and kidney disease, stroke, blindness, hypertension, and even death.

REMEMBER GOD'S LOVE

There is no greater love in the universe than the love God feels for you. No matter what you've done or neglected to do, He loves you more than you could ever know. And He longs to reveal His love to you in every place of emotional need. He wants you to give Him all of the hurts, hidden pain, and disappointments that you've been carrying around. The Bible instructs you to "cast all your care upon Him, because He cares for you" (1 Pet. 5:7, MEV). In Matthew 11:28 Jesus said, "Come to Me" (MEV).

Whether because of nervousness, a lack of comfort, a numb inability to really face your emotional pain, or a hollow sense of aloneness, how often have you relied on filling an empty place in your heart with a piece of pie or a cupcake? Just as with a drug, food can temporarily anesthetize you to the pain of loneliness, abandonment, fear, stress, and emotional pain. It's no wonder the population is literally growing larger. Americans are emotionally hurting from a lack of love. But food cannot truly fill that void.

Have you ever felt that your cravings for certain foods were somehow a guilty reflection of you? Unhealthy food cravings are merely your body's way of signaling you that something is out of whack. From now on commit your cravings to God the moment they occur. He will give you the strength to get through them without overeating, and the grace and wisdom to understand what your body or heart is trying to tell you.

Let your cravings begin a process of bringing your body back into physical and spiritual balance, and with that balance, better health.

One of the main emotional motivators that can send you racing to the refrigerator for comfort is stress. Stress works against you in other ways too. When you are under stress, your body produces a hormone called cortisol, which is similar to cortisone. If you have ever taken cortisone, you are well aware of the side effects. Cortisone causes you to gain weight. Cortisol can have the same effect. When your adrenal glands produce cortisol during periods of high anxiety and stress, it can actually cause your body to gain weight. Therefore, reducing your level of stress can help you lose weight and keep it off, which will improve the condition of your gut.

Chapter 17

LET GO OF ENVY, JEALOUSY, AND ANGER

P ROVERBS 14:30 SAYS, "A calm and undisturbed mind and heart are the life and health of the body, but envy, jealousy, and wrath are like rottenness of the bones" (AMP). This is one of the subtlest yet most common ways the enemy tries to steal our health.

The gut is often referred to as the second brain. Its nerves and cells hold feelings and memory much like those in the brain. Your gut has a neurological network coursing through it. Have you ever felt butterflies in your stomach when you were preparing for a speech or presentation? Have you ever felt your stomach drop when you got bad news or when you ran into that ex-friend from so long ago? Your gut's health is connected to your emotional state of being, so much so that you can experience difficulty digesting food and absorbing its nutrients if you are stressed, angry, bitter, jealous, and more.

The opposite is true as well. If you have a positive disposition, are relaxed and feeling free of negative emotion, you can experience greater benefits from properly digested food. As we have already discovered, when your gut is healthy, your immune system is healthy, and therefore you are able to maintain a better defense against illness and disease. Let's go a little further.

Did you know that your bone marrow manufactures the cells of your immune system? God designed each of us with an automatic health-maintenance system we call the immune system. The immune system guards us against sickness at all times. When a virus, bacteria, fungus, or parasite attacks your body, your immune system goes into action against the invasion. Your very own internal army begins manufacturing and releasing chemicals that destroy the unwanted intruders.

In some cases special antibodies surround the infectious agent and help usher it out of your body. This is why you don't get sick every time you are exposed to these potential disease-causing entities. This is a very good mechanism, since you are exposed to these sorts of pathogens all the time. You are not sick all the time thanks to your immune system—as long as it functions the way God designed it.

Now remember what Proverbs 14:30 said about your bones, the place in your body where your immune system is manufactured. Envy, jealousy, and anger rot your bones. Rotten bones mean rotten bone marrow—and rotten bone marrow means a rotten immune system. In other words, envy, jealousy, and anger set you up for disease! These negative, fear-based emotions are among the most potent stressors your body deals with. And today's medical science has proven time and again that stress is the number one enemy of your immune system.

For example, when you get angry, your blood pressure rises, respiration increases, and nutritional demands and heart rate can skyrocket. Your body goes into survival mode, pumping most of your blood to your muscles. During this state of high alert, your immune system is temporarily neglected—and when you are consuming food in this state you open yourself up to acid reflux, indigestion, and poor absorption that can lead to what we've identified as leaky gut. Perhaps that is why the Bible says not to let the sun go down on your anger (Eph. 4:26).

You need to resolve these negative emotions. When you let them dominate your life, you weaken your immune system. Make a decision right now to not let negative emotions destroy your ability to stay strong against sickness and disease. You can strengthen your immune system by praying today to receive God's forgiveness—and by forgiving others.

Relieving Stress

One of the most common causes of heartburn and indigestion is hypochlorhydria, which is decreased gastric acid secretion or not enough hydrochloric acid. Approximately 50 percent of people over the age of fifty have low stomach acidity; stress accounts for much of this. Your body may be telling you that you are under too much stress if you have any of the following symptoms:

- Difficulty falling asleep
- Not rested when you get up from sleeping
- Physical aches and pains
- Feeling depressed or anxious
- Panic feelings, including your heart racing and perhaps feeling light-headed
- Stomach upset
- Diarrhea

If you can identify four or more of these, you may be experiencing too much stress. Major life traumas such as the death of a spouse, divorce, menopause, and a jail term or probation rank at the top of stressors, followed by the death of a close family member or marriage. Stress can quickly turn a healthy body into an unhealthy body.

Stress can cause a lot of problems for your body, one of which is low stomach acidity—which in turn can cause heartburn and indigestion. Healthy digestion occurs best when you are relaxed and your heart isn't racing. In our fast-paced society too many people work, live, and eat at a crazy pace, which is similar to driving your car all the time with your accelerator to the floor. This ultimately harms your digestive processes. Addressing this situation may require meetings with your physician, spiritual advisor, or a personal counselor to help you address the underlying causes of your acid reflux.

Make a Change Today!

Are you jealous? Most of us have experienced that feeling at least once in our lives. While jealousy seldom improves a relationship, it does harm the person experiencing that emotion. Stress relief expert Lauren E. Miller found that jealousy-induced stress can lead to serious illness, even cancer. She says, "There are many emotions that course through your body during the day that can rapidly increase the stress hormone along with blood pressure in your body, jealousy being one of them."[1]

Harvard Medical School research has shown that 80 percent of disease is stress-related.[2] Jealousy is a high-stress condition. Why is it so stressful? Because like a sinus toothache, jealousy strikes a nerve at our very core: the feeling that we are unworthy, not good enough, or a failure.

God's solution to jealousy is Ephesians 1:6, "To the praise of the glory of His grace, by which He made us accepted in the Beloved" (NKJV). God accepts you, and this reflects your true value. It makes no sense to compare yourself with anyone else. That you are "accepted in the Beloved" means you are loved. Focus your attention on God's love for you, not on how you compare with someone else.

Chapter 18

MENTAL FOG AND ALERTNESS

IN CHAPTER 7 on autoimmune diseases we mentioned Alzheimer's disease as one of the outcomes of inflammation caused by the modern Western diet. Alzheimer's is a degenerative disease in which the nerve cells of the brain deteriorate, resulting in impaired memory, thinking, and behavior. Among its most common symptoms are disorientation, confusion, memory loss, irritability, and reversion to childhood. The disease is progressive, with death occurring about ten years after diagnosis.

Although it takes years to see the outcome, what you eat can incapacitate you mentally. The net effect of foods and an environment full of pesticides, herbicides, and pollution is taking its toll on Americans' bodies—not just on the lungs, blood pressure, or immune system, but also on the nerve and brain cells. Although not always to blame, nutritional deficiencies are a prime cause of Alzheimer's, along with the overuse of prescription drugs. Among other contributing factors are poor circulation, arteriosclerosis, thyroid malfunction, and possible viral connections. Genetic predisposition is present in more than half of the cases.

Granted, everyone shows signs of forgetfulness occasionally, especially with age, so be careful not to confuse misplacing your keys with serious impairment. Still, be aware that the problem of neurological impairment (Alzheimer's disease, dementia, and severe memory loss) is on the rise. In 2014 an estimated 5.2 million Americans had Alzheimer's; two-thirds were women. By 2050 the number of people age 65 and over with the disease may triple.[1] If you or a loved one has concerns, start with a visit to your primary care doctor.

Memory Boosters?

Studies suggest that postmenopausal women who take estrogen replacement therapy (ERT) develop Alzheimer's disease at a lower rate than women who do not. This is because estrogen may help the brain withstand Alzheimer's by promoting the growth and branching of nerve cells in the brain and by improving blood flow and circulation there.[2]

Caution: It is important to note that estrogen increases the risk for breast, uterine, and ovarian cancer over time. Women with a family history of any of these hormone-related cancers should not take estrogen. If you do take estrogen, take natural estrogen, and only after having your hormone levels assayed by saliva or serum (blood work) to verify that a deficiency is present.

In addition to ERT, a study has found that the use of NSAIDs (nonsteroidal anti-inflammatory drugs) such as ibuprofen and naproxen reduced the risk of Alzheimer's disease 30 to 60 percent. This leads researchers to believe that inflammation in the brain may play a part in the disease. Aspirin and acetaminophen were found not to have any positive impact in the study.[3]

In another study that included patients with moderately severe Alzheimer's, Alzheimer's progression was slowed by high doses of vitamin E—as much as 2,000 IU of vitamin E daily. As a result, these patients had a six- to seven-month delay in the progression of the dementia caused by the disease. The normal daily dose of vitamin E is 30 IU. Higher doses should only be taken under the supervision of a health care professional.[4]

Regardless of what the doctor says, recognize that healthy nutritional habits can help overcome the effects of Alzheimer's disease, especially if you make those choices early in life. Start by avoiding red meats and sugar, while eating nuts, eggs, and soy. Choose a largely vegetarian diet and organic foods to avoid harmful substances from pesticides. As part of this plan, eat foods that block aluminum toxicity, such as liver, fish, brown rice, wheat germ, and molasses. Drink spring water only, as fluoridated water increases aluminum absorption. Also, eat avocados, poultry, and low-fat dairy to boost tryptophan levels. Take vitamins, minerals, and nutritional supplements that enhance memory, nourish the brain, and protect brain cells.

Since higher than normal mercury levels have been found in the brains of people with Alzheimer's disease, don't discount mercury exposure—which occurs mainly through dental amalgams—as a potential contributor. Mercury toxicity releases into the brain and affects brain health. If you have any silver amalgam dental fillings, consider having a biological dentist remove them.

DETERMINING SEVERITY

The key to deciding whether memory impairment indicates a serious problem is to determine if it is *progressive*. For example, consider Pete, a businessman in his late fifties. One day sitting at his office desk, he looks around for his favorite fountain pen (again) and wonders, "Why do I keep losing this pen?" A few minutes later Pete finds it in the spot where he had left it. He thinks no more about it until later, when he notices he is forgetting names of acquaintances, and then names of close friends. Finally one day, to his consternation, he gets into his car and realizes he cannot remember the way home.

In the earlier stages of this man's forgetfulness, there was no real cause for alarm. Once it became progressive and he forgot familiar information, the problem became more apparent. To determine the cause, doctors use a standard memory test. They will state three words aloud to the patient—such as *run*, *blue*, and *table*—and then tell the person he or she will be asked to repeat those words later. Whether the patient can complete this task tells the doctor a great deal about the memory centers. Because Alzheimer's affects these areas of the brain first, it is possible to pinpoint potential early onset if the patient fails the test.

Some degree of forgetfulness can be caused by distraction or a lack of attention when the information is given. The distraction prevents the listener from incorporating what he or she heard and moving it into the memory centers. For that reason, doctors will also ask about a patient's childhood. Most early Alzheimer's patients are able to recall childhood memories, but the majority cannot repeat the list of words. So doctors work backward to find out where the degree of forgetfulness begins and determine the level of impairment.

Serious Symptoms

There are certain symptoms neurologists check for regarding a diagnosis of Alzheimer's or serious memory impairment. The following are the most common:

+ Short-term memory loss

    As mentioned previously, when doctors give patients three words to remember and repeat later, the majority with Alzheimer's are unable to remember two of the three.

+ Problems with simple arithmetic

    Alzheimer's patients have great difficulty performing calculations or simple arithmetic in their minds—sums such as two plus five equals seven.

+ Repetition

    If your uncle loves to retell a fishing story, it doesn't mean that he is in the early stages of Alzheimer's. But if someone endlessly repeats details because they can't remember sharing them five minutes earlier, that signals a problem.

+ Getting lost in familiar places

    If a person has taken the same route home from work for ten years, but one day cannot remember which way to go, it is a warning sign.

+ Poor judgment

    Suddenly wearing soiled clothing or forgetting to bathe stems from an impaired mental state. Another example is when a woman continually forgets to turn off the oven or a man leaves the car running in the driveway.

+ Forgetting names

    Forgetting the names of strangers or one-time

acquaintances does not usually signal a significant problem. However, it is serious when a person can't remember the names of a parent, child, relative, or close friend.

Any one of these symptoms may not indicate a crisis, but if more than one manifests along with signs of progressive memory loss, consider getting some help.

NATURAL REMEDIES

Until the early 2000s the medical community believed that once a neuron or nerve cell died—including the cells of the brain—it could never be regenerated or brought back to life. However, scientists have discovered that brain cells, or neurons, can regenerate under the proper conditions. The following natural substances are proven remedies for improving memory function and stopping Alzheimer's progress.

The first is huperzine-A (club moss). When the brain's nerve cells communicate among themselves, they send signals to the body to perform various functions—the heart to beat, the lungs to breathe, or the feet to walk. This communication occurs because of the various chemicals that move in areas between the cells, called synapses. The chemical that communicates memories between these neurons is called *acetylcholine*. As you age, the level of acetylcholine in your brain begins to decrease.

A number of drugs increase the chemical acetylcholine in our brains and thus promote memory, such as Aricept, Cognex, Exelon, and Reminyl. However, they are very expensive and, like all man-made drugs, have side effects.

A natural source of the chemical huperzine-A is synthesized from the club moss plant. It inhibits the enzyme that breaks down acetylcholine in the brain, allowing levels to increase. And it has proven as effective as prescription drugs. The club moss plant has increased memory, thinking ability, focus, and concentration in many Alzheimer's patients. The recommended dosage is 0.1 milligrams daily.

Another natural substance is periwinkle (vinpocetine). For years periwinkle has been used in traditional treatments for cancer because of vincristine. In the early 1980s scientists learned that the vincristine in periwinkle helped with memory loss. This chemical's primary function is causing the blood vessels to widen. This improves memory function by enlarging the blood vessels to the brain, allowing more oxygen and nutrient supply to reach it.

Although the brain only requires about 2 percent of the space within the body, it demands about 20 percent of the oxygen and glucose as its primary energy source. Other cells and tissues are able to utilize either glucose or fat, but the brain requires glucose, which must be delivered through the bloodstream. So, when a natural substance works to cause the blood vessels to the brain to enlarge, it increases the blood supply to the brain. With increased oxygen and glucose levels, memory and concentration will improve as absentmindedness and confusion fade. One milligram daily is the recommended dose.

Other helpful substances are phosphatidylserine (or PS), ginkgo (avoid if on blood thinners), B-vitamins 6 and 12, and vitamin E.

Chapter 19

CAREFUL COOKING AND
MINDFUL EATING

ESEARCHER EDWARD HOWELL devoted nearly his entire life
to researching enzymes. He found that when food is cooked at
temperatures exceeding 118 degrees for thirty minutes, almost
all the enzymes are destroyed. These enzymes are the living part of
the food.[1] When you boil vegetables, the nutrients leach into the water.
By the time the vegetables are tender enough to eat, the mineral and
vitamin content of the water is greater than that of the vegetables! You
have created a dead food from a living food.

If you must boil vegetables, bring the water to a boil first, and then
add your vegetables for a brief time. Do not allow them to soak in the
water. Drain them immediately and serve them. If possible, just quit
boiling vegetables altogether.

Never deep-fry foods. The oils used in deep-frying are usually toxic,
and the meat soaks up these harmful oils like a sponge. However, light
stir-frying in healthy oils is acceptable.

WAVE GOOD-BYE TO THE MICROWAVE

One study found that just six minutes of microwave cooking destroyed
half the vitamin B_{12} in dairy foods and meat, a much higher rate of destruction than other cooking methods.[2] In another test, microwaved broccoli
lost between 87 and 97 percent of several major cancer-protecting antioxidants.[3] I recommend using a convection oven or a toaster oven to heat
up just about anything that you would heat in a microwave oven.

COOKWARE

Here is a list of cookware that is healthy to prepare foods in:

- Glass bakeware and cookware (Pyrex is excellent)
- Ceramic cookware (CorningWare is a recommended brand),
  but throw away if the enamel becomes chipped

+ Stainless steel cookware
+ Anodized aluminum cookware uses an electrochemical anodizing process that seals the aluminum, preventing leaching into the food. This is the *only* acceptable option for aluminum cookware.

Cooking Methods

+ Stir-fry. Use a little bit of organic coconut oil, organic butter, ghee (clarified butter), or macadamia nut oil. Extra-virgin olive oil has a lower smoke point than these oils and will begin to break down when heated over 320 degrees Fahrenheit.
+ Steaming. This is a wonderful way to cook vegetables. Lightly steaming your vegetables causes very little loss of nutrients.
+ Grilling. Use a propane gas grill in place of charcoal or mesquite, which contain dangerous chemicals. Place the meat rack as high as possible, away from the flame. When meat cooks over a flame, fat drips into the fire and turns into steam. The pesticides in the fat char into the meat. Charred meat contains a chemical called benzopyrene, which is a highly carcinogenic substance. Scrape off char. Don't even give it to the dog.
+ Baking or roasting. Drizzle or spritz meats and vegetables with olive oil, sea salt, and freshly ground black pepper. Then roast them in the oven for half an hour, and you have a tasty, healthy alternative to fried foods. Sweet potatoes, tomatoes, and asparagus are especially tasty when roasted this way.

Setting the Atmosphere

The atmosphere at dinnertime should be completely joyful. Turn off the TV. Don't watch sporting events, the news, or suspenseful movies at dinner. Start your meal with a heartfelt blessing. Pause and consider how thankful you are. Then keep the conversation pleasant. Don't use the dinner table as a time to hold court on your children or to bring up troubling topics. Never make dinner a time to reprimand one another or argue. In Leonardo da Vinci's *The Last Supper* you see the disciples laughing, talking, and leaning against Jesus in complete fellowship. That's a good model.

I sometimes hear people yelling and arguing in restaurants. That is the worst way to eat! When you are stressed, you can't digest well. Blood flows away from the digestive tract to the muscles for a fight-or-flight response. This shuts down the digestive juices. Food stays in the stomach longer, causing heartburn and indigestion. Also, the food is not digested properly, leading to bloating, gas, constipation, and even diarrhea.

If you are upset, angry, or in an irritated mood, wait to eat.

Natural Remedies for Heartburn

Heartburn is a burning sensation in the chest that occurs when hydrochloric acid from the stomach backs up into the esophagus. Symptoms include a burning sensation in the stomach and/or chest. If you live with chronic heartburn and indigestion, chances are you are aging faster than normal because your body's energy is reduced, toxins have accumulated, allergic reactions have occurred, and your immune defenses are low. What's more, as people age, digestion weakens because their body produces less stomach acid, meaning you cannot digest proteins well.

Following some simple natural medicine remedies will improve heartburn ailments. As your digestion normalizes, you will notice that almost everything will improve. You will have more energy, sleep better, and feel lighter and more energetic.

To start with, avoid onions, chocolate, citrus fruits, coffee, alcohol, spicy foods, tomato sauce, milk, and soft drinks. On the plus side, eat pineapple, which aids digestion. Digestion is optimal when foods are eaten together that have the same approximate digestion time. To facilitate optimal digestion, follow these guidelines:

- Proteins are eaten alone.
- Vegetables are eaten with grains and legumes.
- Starches and proteins should not be eaten together (although you can eat rice with protein).
- Digestive enzymes taken with a meal will enhance digestion.

Getting back to eating meals together as a family—even if just one or two days a week—is important, especially for children. Sitting down to a meal together, especially dinner, gives parents a chance to reconnect with their children. Even if they're teenagers, you can attempt to spend time with them. The benefits will extend far beyond nutrition. Studies have found that teens who have five or more family dinners per week are three times less likely to try marijuana, two and a half times less likely to smoke cigarettes, and one and a half times less likely to drink alcohol than those who eat with their families less often. Studies also show that teens who eat with their parents are more likely to get better grades and to know that their parents are proud of them.[4]

Healthy Eating Tips

- Chew each bite at least twenty to thirty times, and put your fork down between bites. Your saliva contains special enzymes called *ptyalin* and *amylase*, which digest carbohydrates. Let these enzymes do their work.
- Use your molars to chew. Don't use your canines to eat, as lions and tigers do. They have short digestive tracts and tremendous levels of hydrochloric acid to break down the meat. By contrast, you and I don't produce enough hydrochloric acid to digest half-chewed meat, so it putrefies in the intestines.
- Slow down and enjoy what you are eating. Rushing through a meal causes hydrochloric acid to be suppressed, making digestion difficult. It also encourages you to eat more than

you should. It takes about twenty minutes for your hypo-thalamus, located in your brain, to tell you that you are full. Many people can shovel in thousands of calories before the hypothalamus finally registers "enough."

+ Don't drink cold drinks with food. It dampens and dilutes hydrochloric acid, digestive juices, and enzymes. It's similar to starting a campfire and then pouring water on it. However, a cup of hot organic tea may benefit digestion.

+ Eat the protein portion of your meal first since this stimulates glucagon, which will depress insulin secretion and cause the release of carbohydrates that have been stored in the liver and muscles, which will help prevent low blood sugar.

+ Limit your starches to only one serving per meal. Never eat bread, pasta, potatoes, corn, and different starches together at one meal. This elevates insulin levels. If you feel like having seconds, choose fruits, vegetables, and salads, not more starches.

+ And remember to exercise temperance. Dinner should not be the blowout meal of the day. Eat breakfast like a king, lunch like a prince, and dinner like a pauper. Eat moderate portions and feast instead on conversation and laughter.

Generally your first deep breath toward the end of a meal is a sign that your body is satisfied and that you should stop eating. Continuing to eat after this deep breath regularly will eventually result in weight gain.

Chapter 20

DELICIOUS JUICE, SMOOTHIE, AND LIVING FOOD RECIPES FOR YOUR GUT

YOU ARE WHAT you eat. Now that we have discussed what to eat, how to cook it, and the state of mind you need to derive the maximum benefit from your food, here are fifteen delicious recipes you can incorporate in your daily meal plan that will bring further healing to your lower half.

DIGESTION HELPERS

One of the keys to gut health is improving your digestive system. Here is a recipe for a natural juice drink that will help. Fennel juice is known to aid digestion and relieve gas. Ginger root is also a gas reliever.

> 3 fennel stalks and bulb with fronds
> 1 cucumber, peeled if not organic
> 1 pear
> 1-inch-chunk ginger root
>
> Cut produce to fit your juicer's feed tube. Juice all ingredients and stir. Pour into a glass and drink as soon as possible. Serves 1-2.

In addition, here is a colon cleanser that will improve your gut. Apples are good sources of soluble fiber, which is beneficial for the colon.

> 2 green apples
> 1/2 lemon, peeled if not organic
> 1 handful spinach
> 1 handful parsley
> 2 dark green lettuce leaves
>
> Cut produce to fit your juicer's feed tube. Juice ingredients and stir. Pour into a glass and drink as soon as possible. Serves 1.

CONSTIPATION RELIEF

Constipation problems are a sign of an unhealthy gut. Proper elimination is vital to restoring good health. Try this natural method of curing constipation instead of using an over-the-counter medication or fiber product.

> 2 plums, pitted
> 2 ribs of celery with leaves
> 1 apple
> 1 pear
> 1/2 cucumber, peeled if not organic

Cut produce to fit your juicer's feed tube. Juice ingredients and stir. Pour into a glass and drink as soon as possible. Serves 2.

FIBER-BOOSTING RECIPES

Recipe: Breakfast Cereal

> 1/2 cup Fiber One cereal
> 1/3 cup oat bran

Combine both cereals in a bowl and add fat-free milk.

Recipe: Oat Bran Muffins

> 2 cups oat bran cereal
> 1/4 cup brown sugar, firmly packed
> 2 tsp. baking powder
> 1 cup fat-free (or 1- or 2-percent low-fat) milk
> 3 egg whites, beaten slightly
> 1/4 cup honey
> 2 Tbsp. extra-virgin olive or canola oil

Combine all ingredients. Mix well and pour mixture into 12 muffin cups lined with paper baking liners. Fill muffin cups three-fourths full. Bake at 425 degrees for 15 to 17 minutes.

Beans = fiber

The humble bean is a fantastic way to introduce more fiber into your daily diet. Here are three recipes for preparing beans.

Cooking dried beans

This is one healthy way to cook beans. Rinse a pound of dried beans in a colander and discard any "bad" beans. Place remaining beans in a pot of cold water. Add 1 tablespoon sea salt. Bring beans to a boil, then cover the pot and turn off the heat. Let set overnight. The next morning, cook the beans until they are tender (several hours), following the directions on the bean package.

You can add many ingredients to beans, such as chicken or turkey bones, garlic, onions, celery, tomatoes, and cilantro. Herbs and spices you can add include basil, ground pepper, cumin, oregano, thyme, rosemary, creole seasoning, and other favorites. Dried bean varieties to use include great northern, navy, pinto, lima, black, and butter beans.

Recipe: Pinto Beans Deluxe

4–6 cups cooked pinto beans

1 medium chopped onion

1 16-oz. can stewed tomatoes

1 Tbsp. Mexican-style chili powder

1 handful fresh cilantro

Follow the directions on the dried bean package to cook the beans; just before the beans have finished cooking, add the onion, tomatoes, chili powder, and handful of fresh cilantro.

Recipe: Mediterranean-Style Bean Soup

---

1 Tbsp. extra-virgin olive oil

1 large chopped onion

3 medium peeled and chopped carrots

2 crushed garlic cloves

2 cups dried beans, soaked and drained

8 cups boiling water

1 14-oz. can stewed tomatoes with juice

1 Tbsp. fresh crumbled thyme (or 1 tsp. dried)

2 bay leaves

Approximately 1/4 cup chopped parsley, plus some for garnish

Sea salt and freshly ground black pepper to taste

Croutons for garnish (optional)

Soak the beans overnight, or prepare according to package directions. In a heavy three-quart stock pot, heat the olive oil and sauté the onion, carrots, and garlic until the vegetables are soft but not browned (about 10 minutes). Add the drained beans and boiling water to soup pot; add thyme, bay leaves, and parsley. Cover and cook over low heat 1 to 3 hours, adding water occasionally as needed, or until beans are soft (cooking time varies with type of beans). When beans are soft, add the salt and pepper. For thicker soup, remove about 1 1/2 cups of beans and purée in a food processor or blender. Return to pot. For thinner soup, add hot water. Garnish with chopped parsley or croutons.

INFLAMMATION FIGHTERS

Here are a pair of tonics that will fight the inflammation that can cause problems in your gut area and beyond.

Recipe: Bladder-Healer Tonic

Cranberry juice has been proven in scientific studies to halt bladder infections that can affect gut health. This juice has substances—tannins and hippuric acid—that prevent bacteria from sticking to the bladder wall. Parsley helps decrease inflammation in the bladder. Try this recipe as a tonic for bladder health.

2 organic green apples

1/2 cup fresh or frozen (thawed) cranberries

1 small handful parsley

1 dark green lettuce leaf

1 small lemon, peeled if not organic

Cut produce to fit your juicer's feed tube. Juice 1 apple first. Turn off the machine, add the cranberries, and put the plunger in, then turn the machine on and juice. Wrap parsley in lettuce leaf and juice slowly. Follow with the lemon, and second apple. Stir and pour into a glass; drink as soon as possible. Makes 1 serving.

Recipe: Kidney Tonic

Asparagus is a traditional remedy for bladder and kidney cleansing, and parsley helps to decrease inflammation and irritation in the bladder and urethra. They are also both good diuretics.

    1 handful parsley
    1 dark green lettuce leaf
    8 asparagus stems
    2-3 carrots, scrubbed well, green tops removed, ends trimmed
    1 cucumber, peeled if not organic
    1 medium lemon, washed, or peeled if not organic
    1/2 green apple

Cut produce to fit your juicer's feed tube. Wrap parsley in the lettuce leaf and push through the juicer slowly. Juice all remaining ingredients. Pour into a glass, stir, and drink as soon as possible. Serves 1-2.

More Garlic in Your Diet

Here are three recipes to get more garlic into your diet as a way to improve gut health.

Recipe: Garlic-Lemon Dressing

This dressing is used in eastern Mediterranean countries, both on green salads and on steamed vegetables. This recipe will make 1/4 cup.

    1/2 garlic clove
    1 tsp. sea salt
    1 Tbsp. fresh lemon juice
    3 Tbsp. extra-virgin olive oil
    Freshly ground black pepper to taste

In a clean, dry salad bowl, crush the garlic and salt together with a spoon to make a smooth paste. Add the lemon juice and stir until the salt is dissolved. Add the olive oil and pepper. Mix the dressing well.

Recipe: Garlic Surprise

Here is a healthy gut drink whose taste may surprise you.

1 dark green lettuce leaf
Handful of parsley
1/2 medium cucumber, peeled if not organic
1 garlic clove
3 carrots, scrubbed well, green tops removed, ends trimmed
2 ribs of celery with leaves

Wrap the parsley in the lettuce leaf. Juice the cucumber, the parsley-lettuce wrap, add the garlic, and push through the juicer with the carrots, followed by the celery. Stir and pour into a glass and drink as soon as possible. Serves 1-2.

Recipe: Mediterranean Spinach Enchiladas

1 1/2 cups nonfat chicken broth
1 cup diced mild canned green chili peppers
2 diced tomatoes
2 Tbsp. finely chopped onions
2 cloves minced garlic
2 Tbsp. cornstarch
2 Tbsp. water
1 1/4 lb. fresh chopped spinach
8 corn tortillas

In a 2-quart saucepan, combine the broth, chili peppers, tomatoes, onions, and garlic. Bring to a boil. Simmer over low heat for 15 minutes. In a small bowl, combine the cornstarch and water. Add to the broth and continue cooking, stirring as the mixture cooks until it thickens. Remove from the heat.

While the sauce is cooking, steam the spinach for 5 minutes. Coat a 9- by 13-inch baking dish with a no-cholesterol, no-stick cooking spray. Divide the spinach equally among the tortillas and roll, placing a single layer of enchiladas in the baking dish with the open side down. Top with the tomato mixture. Bake at 400 degrees for 10 minutes. This tasty dish will make a complete meal when served with a salad.

RECIPE: Happy Liver Cleansing Cocktail

Chapter 14 reviews healthy gut detoxes. Here is another that includes beets, which are traditionally used to cleanse the liver. If you have a sugar sensitivity such as diabetes or hypoglycemia, always dilute beet and carrot juice with cucumber and other greens. You may only be able to juice very small portions of beet and carrot.

    3 carrots, scrubbed well, tops removed, ends trimmed
    1 cucumber, peeled if not organic
    1 beet with stem and leaves, scrubbed well
    2 ribs of celery with leaves
    1 handful parsley
    1 dark green lettuce leaf
    1-2-inch-chunk ginger root, scrubbed or peeled if old
    1/2 lemon, peeled if not organic

Cut produce to fit your juicer's feed tube. Juice all ingredients and stir. Pour into a glass and drink as soon as possible. Serves 1-2.

MOOD LIFTERS

Recipe: Antianxiety Cocktail

If you are prone to anxiety attacks or find yourself with gut diseases related to emotional upheaval, here is a mixture that can help you calm down. Magnesium is known as "nature's valium." Include plenty of magnesium-rich veggies in fresh-squeezed juices, such as beet leaves, spinach, parsley, dandelion greens, broccoli, cauliflower, carrots, and celery.

    1 handful spinach
    1 dark green lettuce leaf

3-4 carrots, scrubbed well, tops removed, ends trimmed

2 ribs of celery with leaves

1 broccoli stem

1 lemon, peeled if not organic

Cut produce to fit your juicer's feed tube. Wrap the spinach in the lettuce leaf and push through the juicer slowly. Juice all remaining ingredients and stir. Pour into a glass and drink as soon as possible. Serves 1.

Recipe: Depression Kicker

If emotional upset is plaguing your gut and threatening to turn into depression, you may lack healthy sodium levels in your diet. Sodium deficiency actually creates symptoms that resemble depression. However, table salt is not a good choice; use only Celtic sea salt or Himalayan salt. You can juice up plenty of sodium-rich vegetables such as celery, chard, beet greens, and spinach to create this drink that can help fight depression.

1 handful spinach

1-2 chard leaves

4 ribs of celery with leaves

1 green apple

1 medium lemon, peeled if not organic

Cut produce to fit your juicer's feed tube. Wrap spinach in chard and push through the juicer slowly. Juice all remaining ingredients and stir. Pour into a glass and drink as soon as possible. Serves 1-2.

Recipe: Allergy Remedies

One of the signs of an unhealthy gut is problems with food and other allergies. Following are two recipes that utilize natural sources to combat allergies. The first relies on the power of parsley, a known "folk remedy" for allergy attacks.

1 large bunch of parsley

1/4-1/2 small or medium lemon washed, or peeled if not organic

2-3 carrots, scrubbed well, tops removed, ends trimmed

2 ribs of celery with leaves

1 cucumber, peeled if not organic

Cut produce to fit your juicer's feed tube. Bunch up parsley and add to the juicer before turning it on. Then add lemon and place the plunger in place. Turn on the machine and juice remaining ingredients. Stir, and pour into a glass. Drink as soon as possible. Serves 1.

The second recipe uses the humble radish, another traditional remedy for asthma.

5 carrots, scrubbed well, green tops removed, ends trimmed

5–6 radishes with leaves

1 green apple

1/2 lemon, peeled if not organic

Juice all ingredients. Stir the juice and pour into a glass. Serve at room temperature or chilled, as desired. Serves 1.

Recipe: Weight-Loss Buddy

Chapter 8 mentions the Jerusalem artichoke as one of the superfoods that will promote gut health. Jerusalem artichoke juice combined with carrot and beet is a traditional remedy for satisfying cravings for sweets and junk food, two items that are bad for your gut. The key with this remedy is to sip it slowly when you get a craving for high-fat or high-carb foods.

3–4 carrots, scrubbed well, tops removed, ends trimmed

1 Jerusalem artichoke, scrubbed well

1 cucumber, peeled if not organic

1 lemon, peeled if not organic

1/2 small beet, scrubbed well, with stems and leaves

Cut produce to fit your juicer's feed tube. Juice ingredients and stir. Pour into a glass and drink as soon as possible. Serves 1–2.

Recipe: Antiaging Rejuvenator

If gut problems are causing signs of aging, try eating more cucumbers and bell peppers. These are good sources of the trace mineral silicon, which is recommended to firm up the skin. In studies, silicon has been shown to reduce signs of aging by improving thickness of skin and reducing wrinkles. Here is a good antiaging drink.

1 cucumber, peeled if not organic

1 parsnip

2–3 carrots, scrubbed well, tops removed, ends trimmed

1/2 lemon, peeled

1/4 green bell pepper

Cut produce to fit your juicer's feed tube. Juice ingredients and stir. Pour into a glass and drink as soon as possible. Serves 1–2.

Chapter 21

CHECK YOURSELF

A NY TIME ADVOCATES raise the idea of using natural foods, supplements, and other methods to address various health issues, people always want to know: "What about seeing a doctor? Does eating natural foods mean I will never have to go to a physician?" Not necessarily. After all, the Bible calls Luke, who wrote the Gospel of Luke and the Book of Acts, "the beloved physician" (Col. 4:14, MEV). Christ's followers see Jesus as the Great Physician who heals all diseases, whether that involves spirit, soul, or body. If you are struggling with such problems as leaky gut syndrome, irritable bowel syndrome, or digestive upsets that keep you up at night, seeing a doctor is a wise course of action.

Still, before consulting any kind of physician, it is a good idea to talk with God and search the Bible for verses that address your situation. Scripture contains promises that are eternal and offer great hope. Yet approaching the Great Physician is often the last thing that comes to people's minds when it ought to be the first thing on your list.

As you contemplate your course of action, don't overlook the help available from three other physicians: Dr. Diet, Dr. Quiet, and Dr. Merryman.

Dr. Diet will tell you to eat the foods God created, because as the old saying goes, "You are what you eat" (you are what you ate too). Your body is constantly changing—literally making itself new out of the foods you have eaten. For instance, every twenty-eight to forty-five days you have a brand-new skin. Your body "sheds" an astonishing forty pounds of dust over your lifetime in the form of skin particles (dander or dandruff) as your skin becomes new. Every six weeks you have a brand-new liver. It only takes three to five days for your stomach lining to be renewed (because of the high acid content, the cells are exchanged quickly). In a twelve-month period 98 percent of your atoms and molecules are replaced, all manufactured from the foods you consume.

Dr. Quiet will tell you to relax the way God modeled—and instructed—when He instituted a Sabbath day of rest. The Bible promises, "A calm and undisturbed mind and heart are the life and health of the body" (Prov. 14:30, AMP). It is healthy to stay calm and relaxed. Practice more than stress management; practice stress elimination by casting all your cares on the One who cares for you (1 Pet. 5:7). Get the rest and exercise you need to rejuvenate body, soul, and spirit, as Jesus did.

Dr. Merryman will quote Proverbs 17:22, "A merry heart does good like a medicine" (MEV). Likewise, Proverbs 15:30 says, "A cheerful look brings joy to the heart; good news makes for good health" (NLT). Put simply, happier people are healthier people. There is a reason the apostle Paul advised, "Friends, I'd say you'll do best by filling your minds and meditating on things true, noble, reputable, authentic, compelling, gracious—the best, not the worst; the beautiful, not the ugly; things to praise, not things to curse" (Phil. 4:8, THE MESSAGE). On the other hand, Proverbs 14:30 warns us that "envy, jealousy, and wrath are like rottenness of the bones" (AMP).

The latter is much too high a price to pay for harboring negative emotions. As mentioned earlier in this book, there are potential links between emotional uproar and gut health. When it comes to improving yours, get rid of such junk in your trunk as negative emotions, anger, holding grudges toward others, and anxiety.

SELF-CHECK HEALTH TEST

Here is a gut health check that you can do yourself. Answer these questions truthfully:

+ Do you handle stress properly? Do you know how to release the pressures that aggravate your condition, and cast your cares on God?
+ Do you always get enough sleep, which has been mentioned several times as an important element of good gut health?
+ Do you follow a consistent exercise program to improve your digestive and other systems? ("Yes" means you *are* following it, not that you *plan* to follow it!)
+ Are fresh fruits on your daily menu?

+ Are fresh vegetables on your daily menu? (French fries don't count!)

+ Are whole grains a staple of your diet? Do you typically avoid SAD—the standard American diet—that is full of processed foods?

+ When you have a choice, do you choose white meat over other meats? Do you choose lean cuts? (Remember, non-organic, fat-filled red meats help clog your colon.)

+ Do you drink at least eight glasses of pure water daily? And, do you also avoid alcohol, soft drinks, coffee, and other unhealthy beverages?

If you cannot answer affirmatively to each question, take heart. You can start putting these keys into practice immediately and plant the seeds of better health habits today.

While you practice good physical habits, practice the principles of spiritual health. Ever hear the adage "You reap what you sow"? That is true because it comes straight from the pages of Scripture: "Whatever a man sows, that will he also reap" (Gal. 6:7, MEV). Nowhere is this truer than in the area of health. You can take simple, positive steps every day to reap the good health promised in God's Word.

Don't hang a long list of "don'ts" on your refrigerator and make a long face every time you look at them (or try *not* to look at them). It can be discouraging to keep thinking about how far you have to go and about all the things you will have to deny yourself to get there. Instead, concentrate on the good things you can do every day that will help you gain ground. Be encouraged and smile when you think of how you *get to* do healthy things instead of *having to* do them. Thank God every morning for the energy to get up and get moving. If your gut health isn't good yet, thank God that you can take one step today in that direction.

Remember that God isn't in the business of *de-stressing*, He's in the business of *no stressing*. He intends your days to be a taste of heaven on earth, something to be enjoyed instead of endured. Get outside every day and take advantage of the fresh air and sunshine He created to give you good health and pleasure.

SEEING THE DOCTOR

As for human doctors, there are appropriate times to pay them a visit. If someone in your family requires a couple stitches, for example, you probably don't want to try handling that at home. Likewise, if the consequences of an upset stomach, constipation, or a clogged colon make your days and nights miserable, you will want to consult an expert on ways to address the problem. Remember, the best way to approach good health is like the director of a stage play. You ultimately make the decisions affecting numerous aspects of the play, but all around you are assistants, stage managers, and other advisors to help carry out the production. Your primary care doctor and various specialists are there to help you produce optimal health.

After all, as we mentioned earlier in this chapter, Proverbs says a merry heart does good *like a medicine*. That implies that medicine does some good. However, as we have reviewed in previous chapters, medicine in the form of natural remedies is safer than manufactured drugs. Many drugs manufactured today can be poisonous to your body and have nasty side effects. It is wise to find a physician who is judicious in what he or she prescribes.

You also want to choose a physician who emphasizes nutrition and living a healthy lifestyle, not someone who concentrates on treating what ails you after the fact and typically turns to prescriptions. Any good physician knows the truth that an ounce of prevention is worth a pound of cure.

Doctors and medicines are sometimes a huge blessing. When you or someone you love suffers a traumatic injury or is involved in an accident, you want a skilled physician on duty in the emergency room. However, when it comes to day-to-day health, you will live longer, look younger, and need less medical attention if you will live by healthy principles. The ideal is to only see the inside of your doctor's office when it's time for a check-up or a short-term, specialized treatment.

NOTES
Chapter 1—Gluten-Free Zone

1. William Davis, *Wheat Belly* (New York: Rodale, 2011), 14.
2. H. C. Broeck, H. C. de Jong, E. M. Salentijn, et al., "Presence of Celiac Disease Epitopes in Modern and Old Hexaploid Wheat Varieties: Wheat Breeding May Have Contributed to Increased Prevalence of Celiac Disease," *Theoretical and Applied Genetics* 121, no. 8 (November 2010): 1527-1539, as referenced in Davis, *Wheat Belly*, 26.
3. Davis, *Wheat Belly*, 35.
4. Ibid., 36, 53–54.
5. Ibid., 45.
6. Linda Page, *Healthy Healing*, 11th ed. (N.p.: Traditional Wisdom, Inc., 2000).

Chapter 2—Probiotics

1. James F. Balch and Phyllis Balch, *Prescription for Nutritional Healing* (Garden City, NY: Avery Publishing Group, 1997).

Chapter 4—Treating IBS

1. St. John's Wort, Wholehealthmd.com: www.wholehealth.com/refshelf (accessed October 22, 2002).

Chapter 5—Fiber and Regularity

1. J. A. Marlett, M. I. McBurney, J. L. Slavin, and American Dietetic Association, "Position of the American Dietetic Association: Health Implications of Dietary Fiber," *Journal of the American Dietetic Association* 102, no. 7 (2002): 993-1000.
2. N. C. Howarth, E. Saltzman, and S. B. Roberts, "Dietary Fiber and Weight Regulation," *Nutrition Review* 59, no. 5 (2001): 129-138.
3. Page, *Healthy Healing*, D371.

Chapter 6—Inflammation

1. Page, *Healthy Healing*, C356.
2. "The World's Healthiest Foods: Chili Pepper, Dried," George Mateljan Foundation, http://www.whfoods.com/genpage.php?tname=foodspice&dbid=29 (accessed May 25, 2012).
3. Page, *Healthy Healing*, C360.

Chapter 7—The Autoimmune Collection

1. "Mercury Contamination in Fish: A Guide to Staying Healthy and Fighting Back," Natural Resources Defense Council, http://www.nrdc.org/health/effects/mercury/guide.asp (accessed May 1, 2013).

Chapter 8 —Superfoods for the Gut

1. "9 Reasons to 'Eat Your Radishes'!" *Full Circle*, May 14, 2012, http://www.full circle.com/goodfoodlife/2012/05/14/9-reasons-to-eat-your-radishes/.

2. "The World's Healthiest Foods: Leeks," George Mateljan Foundation, http://www.whfoods.com/genpage.php?tname=foodspice&dbid=26 (accessed February 27, 2015); Joseph Mercola, "Why Leeks Are Good for You," Mercola.com, February 8, 2014, http://articles.mercola.com/sites/articles/archive/2014/02/08/leeks-benefits.aspx.

3. Diana Herrington, "10 Benefits of Carrots: The Crunchy Powerfood," Care 2, October 26, 2011, http://www.care2.com/greenliving/10-benefits-of-carrots.html.

4. Cheryl Forberg, "5 Powerful Health Benefits of Asparagus You Probably Didn't Know," Eating Well, April 11, 2011, http://www.eatingwell.com/blogs/health_blog/5_powerful_health_benefits_of_asparagus_you_probably_didn_t_know.

5. "Jerusalem Artichoke Nutrition Facts," Power Your Diet, http://www.nutrition-and-you.com/jerusalem-artichoke.html (accessed February 27, 2015); see also Jessica Bruso, "Health Benefits of Jerusalem Artichokes," LiveStrong.com, February 18, 2014, http://www.livestrong.com/article/374796-health-benefits-of-jerusalem-artichokes/.

6. "What Is Jicama (Yambean) Good For?" Mercola.com, http://foodfacts.mercola.com/jicama.html (accessed February 27, 2015); "Jicama (Yam Bean) Nutrition Facts, Power Your Diet, www.nutrition-and-you.com/jicama.html (accessed February 27, 2015).

Chapter 9—Vitamins

1. *The World's Greatest Treasury of Health Secrets*, ed. Boardline, Inc. (Greenwich, CT: Bottomline Books, 2002), 272.

2. "Researchers Report Vitamin # Protects Key Proteins From Damage Due to Aging," Arizona Health Sciences Center, University of Arizona (May 28, 1996), www.ahsc.arizona.edu/opa/news/may96/kay.htm (accessed October 22, 2002).

Chapter 11—Exercise

1. "How Much Physical Activity Do Adults Need?", Centers for Disease Control and Prevention, December 1, 2011, http://www.cdc.gov/physicalactivity/everyone/guidelines/adults.html (accessed March 26, 2013).

2. K. N. Boutelle and D. S. Kirschenbaum, "Further Support for Consistent Self-Monitoring as a Vital Component of Successful Weight Control," *Obesity Research* 6, no. 3 (May 1998): 219-224, http://www.ncbi.nlm.nih.gov/pubmed/9618126 (accessed March 21, 2013).

Chapter 13—Acid Reflux

1. M. H. Pittler and E. Ernst, "Peppermint Oil for Irritable Bowel Syndrome: A Critical Review and Metaanalysis," *The American Journal of Gastroenterology* 93(7) (1998): 1131-1135; J. H. Liu et al., "Enteric-Coated Peppermint Oil Capsules in the Treatment of Irritable Bowel Syndrome: A Prospective, Randomized Trial," *Journal of Gastroenterology* 32 (1997): 765-768; M. J. Dew, B. K. Evans and J. Rhodes, "Peppermint Oil for the Irritable Bowel Syndrome: A Multicenter Trial," *Br J Clin Pract* 38 (1984): 394-398.

Chapter 15—Food Sensitivities

1. Page, *Healthy Healing*, 319.

Chapter 16—End Emotional Eating

1. National Diabetes Statistics: General Information and National Estimates on Diabetes in the United States, 2000, NIH Publication No. 02-3892 (March 2002).

Chapter 17—Let Go of Envy, Jealousy, and Anger

1. "Jealousy Paralyzes Creativity, Productivity, and Relationships, Says Stress Relief Expert Lauren E. Miller," PR Newswire, July 12, 2011, http://www.prnewswire.com/news-releases/jealousy-paralyzes-creativityproductivity-and-relationships-says-stress-relief-expert-lauren-e-miller-125405253.html (accessed November 11, 2012).
2. Ibid.

Chapter 18—Mental Fog and Alertness

1. "Alzheimer's Facts and Figures," Alzheimer's Association, http://www.alz.org/alzheimers_disease_facts_and_figures.asp (accessed November 3, 2014).
2. "Estrogen May Delay Alzheimer's Onset in Postmenopausal Women," *Columbia University Record* 22 (September 13, 1996), www.columbia.edu/cu/1996/0913/d.html (accessed October 22, 2002).
3. "Anti-Inflammatories Reduce Risks of Alzheimer's," *Johns Hopkins Gazette* (March 17, 1997), www.jhu.edu/~gazette/janmar97/mar1797/briefs.html (accessed October 22, 2002).
4. Mary Sano, et al., "A Controlled Trial of Selegiline, Alpha-Tocopherol, or Both as Treatment for Alzheimer's Disease," *New England Journal of Medicine* 336 (April 24, 1997): 1216-1222, www.content.nejm.org (accessed October 11, 2002).

Chapter 19—Careful Cooking and Mindful Eating

1. "What Are Enzymes?" Healthy Alternatives, Healthy Reflections: The Function of Enzymes in Nutrition, http://www.healthyalternativesinc.com/enzymes.htm (accessed September 9, 2008).

2. Janet Raloff, "Microwaves Bedevil a B Vitamin—Research Indicates Overcooking and Microwaving Meat and Dairy Foods Inactivate Vitamin B12—Brief Article," *Science News* 153, February 14, 1998, http://www.findarticles.com/p/articles/mi_m1200/is_n7_v153/ai_20346932 (accessed September 9, 2008).

3. B. H. Blanc and H. U. Hertel, "Comparative Study of Food Prepared Conventionally and in the Microwave Oven," published by Raum & Zelt, 1992, in *Journal of the Science of Food and Agriculture* 3, no. 2 (2003): 43.

4. "Casa and TV Land/Nick at Nite Report Shows Frequent Family Dinners Cut Teens' Substance Abuse Risk in Half," National Center on Addiction and Substance Abuse, press release, September 13, 2005, http://www.casacolumbia.org/absolutenm/templates/PressReleases.aspx?articleid=405&zoneid=64 (accessed September 9, 2008).

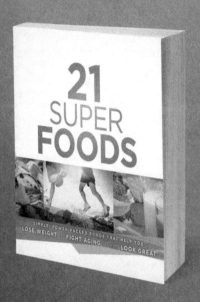

Ignite Your SPIRITUAL HEALTH with these FREE Newsletters

CHARISMA HEALTH
Get information and news on health-related topics and studies, and tips for healthy living.

POWER UP! FOR WOMEN
Receive encouraging teachings that will empower you for a Spirit-filled life.

CHARISMA MAGAZINE NEWSLETTER
Get top-trending articles, Christian teachings, entertainment reviews, videos and more.

CHARISMA NEWS WEEKLY
Get the latest breaking news from an evangelical perspective every Monday.

SIGN UP AT:
nl.charismamag.com

CHARISMA MEDIA